the 8-week blood sugar diet recipe book

Disclaimer:
This publication contains the opinions and ideas of its authors. It is intended to provide helpful and informative material on the subjects addressed in the publication. It is not intended as and should not be relied upon as medical advice. It is sold with the understanding that the authors and publisher are not engaged in rendering medical, health, or any other kind of personal or professional services in the book. The reader should consult his or her medical, health, or other competent professional before adopting any of the suggestions in this book or drawing inferences from it. The authors and publisher specifically disclaim all responsibility for any liability, loss, or risk, personal or otherwise, which is incurred as a consequence, directly or indirectly, of the use and applications of any of the contents of this book. If you have underlying health problems, or have any doubts about the information contained in this book, you should contact a qualified medical, dietary, or other appropriate professional.

Caution – discuss your diet plans with your doctor if any of the following apply:
You have a history of eating disorders
You are on insulin or a diabetic medication other than metformin – you may need to plan how you reduce your medication to avoid too fast a drop in blood sugar
You are on blood pressure tablets – you may have to reduce or come off them
You have moderate or severe retinopathy – you should have an extra screening within six months of reducing or reversing the diabetes
You have a significant psychiatric disorder
You are taking warfarin
You have epilepsy
You have a significant medical condition

Don't go on the diet if:
You are under 18
Your BMI is below 21
You are pregnant or breastfeeding
You are recovering from surgery, are unwell or you are generally frail

Published in 2016 by Short Books
Unit 316
ScreenWorks,
22 Highbury Grove
N5 2ER

20

Copyright © Parenting Matters Ltd
Photographs copyright © Joe Sarah

Page design by Andrew Smith
Cover design and front cover photo by Smith & Gilmour

Clare Bailey has asserted her right under the Copyright, Designs and Patents Act 1988 to be identified as the author of this work. All rights reserved. No part of this publication may be reproduced, stored in a retrieval system or transmitted in any form, or by any means (electronic, mechanical, or otherwise) without the prior written permission of both the copyright owners and the publisher.

A CIP catalogue record for this book is available from the British Library.

Printed in Italy by L.E.G.O. SpA

ISBN: 978-1-78072-293-1

the 8-week blood sugar diet recipe book

DR CLARE BAILEY

with DR SARAH SCHENKER

Photography by Joe Sarah

Contents

Foreword by Dr Michael Mosley page 7

Introduction by Dr Clare Bailey page 9

About the 8-Week Blood Sugar Diet page 12

Breakfast and Brunch page 24

Quick Lunches, Smart Snacks page 46

Easy Weekday Suppers page 78

Main Meals page 120

Veg Sides page 156

Occasional Treats page 178

Swaps and Tips page 196

8-Week Meal Planner page 200

Foreword by Dr Michael Mosley

On my first day at medical school I sat nervously with a hundred other students in a huge lecture theatre while the Dean gave his usual introductory talk. It was a long time ago but I can remember two things he said. Firstly, based on previous experience, he predicted that four of us in the room would marry. He was right: I met my wife that day (more about her later). The other memorable thing he said was that, while we would learn an enormous amount during our medical training, in time much of it would become out of date. Which is why it is so important for doctors (and the rest of us) to try and keep up with the latest science.

I was mindful of this when, in 2012, I went to see my GP with a minor complaint, had a routine blood test and discovered that I was a type 2 diabetic. I was told that I should start on medication. But I wasn't convinced that my only option was to spend a lifetime on drugs. So I started researching alternative approaches.

I came across something called 'intermittent fasting' and, the more I dug, the more interesting it looked. I finally decided to make a documentary about intermittent fasting for the BBC science series, *Horizon*, with myself as the subject.

In the course of making the documentary I put myself on what I called a '5:2 diet', whereby you eat normally five days a week and cut your calories down to around 600 calories for two days. On this diet I lost 9kg in 12 weeks and my blood sugar levels went back to normal. I later co-wrote a book, *The Fast Diet*, which became an international bestseller.

That book was not, however, aimed at diabetics and I wondered at the time why losing the weight had produced such a dramatic impact on my blood sugar levels. Then, in 2015, I met up with Professor Roy Taylor of Newcastle University, one of Europe's leading diabetes experts.

It's been known for some time that too much fat around your middle (so-called visceral fat) greatly increases your risk of diabetes, heart disease and high blood pressure. Our rapidly expanding waists have been a major driver behind the huge rise in rates of type 2 diabetes in recent times. Ideally, your waist (measured round your tummy button) should be less than half your height. In other words, if you are 1.8m tall, your waist should be less than 90cm.

Visceral fat is particularly bad for you because it clogs up your liver and your pancreas (the organ that produces the hormone insulin, which regulates blood sugar levels). Once this happens you are on the path to becoming a diabetic.

The good news, however, is that this is not inevitable. You can do something to both prevent and reverse type 2 diabetes.

Professor Taylor told me he and his team had shown that, if you can reduce your body weight by 10-15%, this shrinks the visceral fat, unclogs your liver and pancreas and, in the majority of diabetic patients, enables them to come off their medication.

Meanwhile, if you are a prediabetic (i.e. you have raised blood sugars but are not yet in the diabetic range) then a 10% reduction in body weight will cut your chance of becoming diabetic by an amazing 90%!

Professor Taylor also surprised me by saying that one of the most effective ways to lose weight and keep it off is through a rapid weight-loss diet. I'd always believed that it's better to lose weight slowly and steadily, but this isn't what the latest science shows.

In clinical trials Professor Taylor's team have shown that going on a programme of 800 calories a day for 8 weeks produces average weight loss of 14kg and reversal of type 2 diabetes in the majority of patients.

His work formed the basis of my most recent book, *The 8-Week Blood Sugar Diet*, and is a founding principle of this companion recipe book.

Although it sounds challenging, most people who have tried the 8-Week Blood Sugar Diet have found it easier than conventional dieting and much more rewarding. Carole, for example, wrote to me to say, *'Having followed the regime in your book I have lost 2.5 stone (16kg) and I no longer have diabetes. I have gone from dress size 14/16 to 10/12. My husband, who was 16st, has lost over 3.5 stone (20kg). It has been life-changing and now that we are eating differently I think my taste buds have changed. I find so much more flavour in food.'*

As Carole hints, it isn't just about cutting your calories, it is also about changing what you eat. I keep my weight off and my blood sugar levels down by minimising sugary and starchy carbs and instead eating a low-carb, Mediterranean-style diet. This is one which is rich in vegetables, fruit, fish, meat, nuts and olive oil – and which allows the occasional glass of wine and chocolate, just not the bread, pasta and potatoes. It's the approach that informs the recipes in this book, which were created by Dr Clare Bailey and Dr Sarah Schenker.

Sarah is a registered dietitian and nutritionist. We've worked together on a number of previous books. I rate her highly.

I am also a big fan of Dr Clare Bailey, a GP who just happens to be my wife. As I mentioned earlier we met at medical school and ever since I've known her she has been passionate about food. She is one of those annoying people who stays slim, seemingly without effort. Her secret is that she rarely snacks and she has always enjoyed a Mediterranean style of eating.

She loves trying different ingredients, different combinations, but she also wanted to produce recipes that are not too complicated or expensive. As a family we have greatly enjoyed testing and tasting the recipes in this book.

Clare's motivation for writing it comes from the fact that as a doctor she has seen so many of her patients do well using the 8-Week Blood Sugar Diet approach. This includes Cassie, an insulin-dependent diabetic who lost 30kg on the diet and who managed to not only come off all medication but also improve her PCOS (polycystic ovary syndrome). After several years of trying, Cassie recently got pregnant and gave birth to twins.

The joy of this diet is that it is extremely flexible. We are all different and have different needs. So, though many people will opt for the intensive 800-calorie approach to achieve the greatest impact and quickest result, you can go more gently. I know people who have started off consuming 800 calories every day, then moved to a slightly more relaxed regime of 800 calories five days a week. Some do the diet two days a week; others have simply changed to the low-blood-sugar way of eating, watching their carb intake, reducing portion sizes but not constantly counting calories. As Lisa recently wrote, *'If you can't cope with 800 I would just up it a little. My mum has lost 8lb and as she is inactive that's brilliant. Her blood sugar is more stable than ever and she's looking great. Give it a go, it could change your life!'*

So, do you want to lose weight, improve your health and get your blood sugars under control? Do you want to do this while eating tasty, filling food? If so, you are in the right place. To eat and to live. That is what this book is all about.

Introduction by Dr Clare Bailey

'Jack Sprat could eat no fat. His wife could eat no lean.

And so between them both, you see, they licked the platter clean'

Michael and I used to be like Jack Sprat and his wife. Twenty years ago, worried about his health, Michael followed standard dietary advice and cut down on fat. I, however, continued to eat what I liked, a diet which included its fair share of fats. Over the next decade he expanded around the middle and developed type 2 diabetes. And I, conversely, seemed to maintain a steady weight. Perhaps the dietary advice we'd been given was wrong?

Well, yes, as it turned out. Cutting out fat, as we now know, both deprives us of a key source of nutrients and tends to lead to an increase in the consumption of other, more pernicious things, like refined carbohydrates. This is just one of the dietary misconceptions that Michael has highlighted in the course of his research into fasting and weight loss. Most recently, in his book *The 8-Week Blood Sugar Diet* he has drawn on new evidence to transform the way we think about food.

Before Michael started his research, as a GP I would typically have told a newly diagnosed type 2 diabetic that they should go on a low-fat diet, cut down on sugar and try to lose some weight. Unfortunately, because this rarely worked, the next step was usually medication.

These days my approach is very different. When I see someone with raised blood sugars I start by explaining that much of the dietary advice we've been giving them for the last few decades has been unhelpful and that there's a lot of science which supports a new approach, involving rapid weight loss as a means of reducing and controlling blood sugar levels. I tell them that once they move away from basing their diet on starchy carbohydrates and sugars they will find that they no longer feel hungry all the time; that their body's natural feedback mechanisms will kick back into action to switch off hunger signals and tell them when they are full.

At this point they normally look hugely relieved. Most, though not all, are then keen to give it a go and those who persist with the Blood Sugar Diet typically see impressive reductions in blood sugar levels within a matter of weeks. They also see significant weight loss and a reduction in waist circumference, often around 5-10cm.

For any of you who have not read Michael's book, *The 8-Week Blood Sugar Diet* sets out a bold and radical programme that involves you sticking to around 800 calories a day for up to 8 weeks. This intensive approach is the fastest way to see change, and the recipes in this book have been designed with that goal in mind. Your calorie intake can be averaged out over the week so it's fine to go up to 900 on some days and down to 700 on others. It does not have to be absolutely exact. All the calorie counts in the recipes here are calculated for a single portion, and, in the spirit of pragmatism, we have rounded them to the nearest 10.

As Michael pointed out in his foreword, the recipes are all based on a Mediterranean style of eating because this has the most rigorous scientific backing when it comes to losing weight and improving blood sugar levels. The other really important thing is that numerous studies have shown that people find this approach satisfying and sustainable, and so you are far more likely to stick to it than to a conventional low-fat diet.

Over the past few years, we have made a conscious effort at home to shift towards a lower-carbohydrate, higher-fat diet, one rich in olive oil, fish, nuts, fruit and vegetables, as well as lots of delicious things that down the years we have been told to avoid, such as full-fat yoghurt and eggs. I love this sort of food and I have thoroughly enjoyed putting the theory behind the diet into practice – developing the recipes for this book.

I hope you will enjoy them too. I have been much cheered by the feedback from my patients, many of whom say that it's the first diet they've felt they can stick to.

No one diet is going to suit everyone. So if you find that 800 calories a day, every day, is too tough to sustain, then, as Michael recommends, you could try the gentler 5:2 approach in which you eat 800 calories two days a week.

On the other five days you should follow a Mediterranean-style way of eating, but without strictly counting calories. This can be done using the recipes in this book, often by simply doubling portion sizes and adding extras to some of your meals such as an additional salad or portion of vegetables or a couple of tablespoons of lentils, beans, bulgar wheat or quinoa. You might add more nuts, seeds, wholegrains, and the occasional piece of wholegrain bread. You won't reach your goals quite as fast with this approach, but it is still effective.

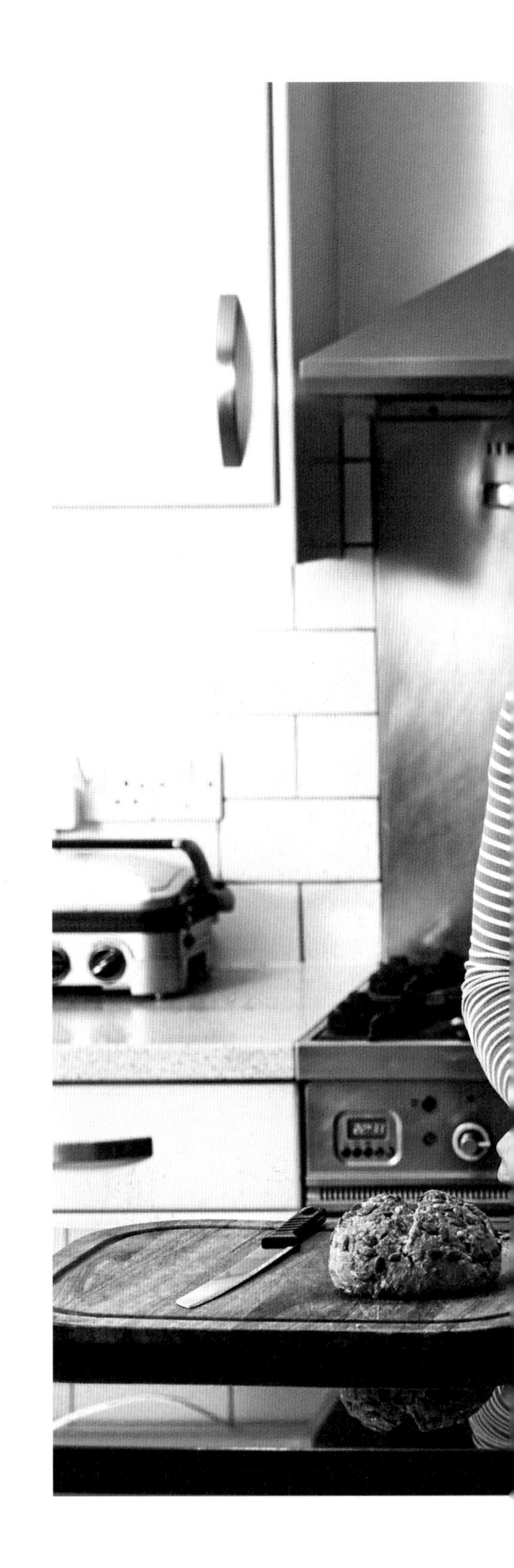

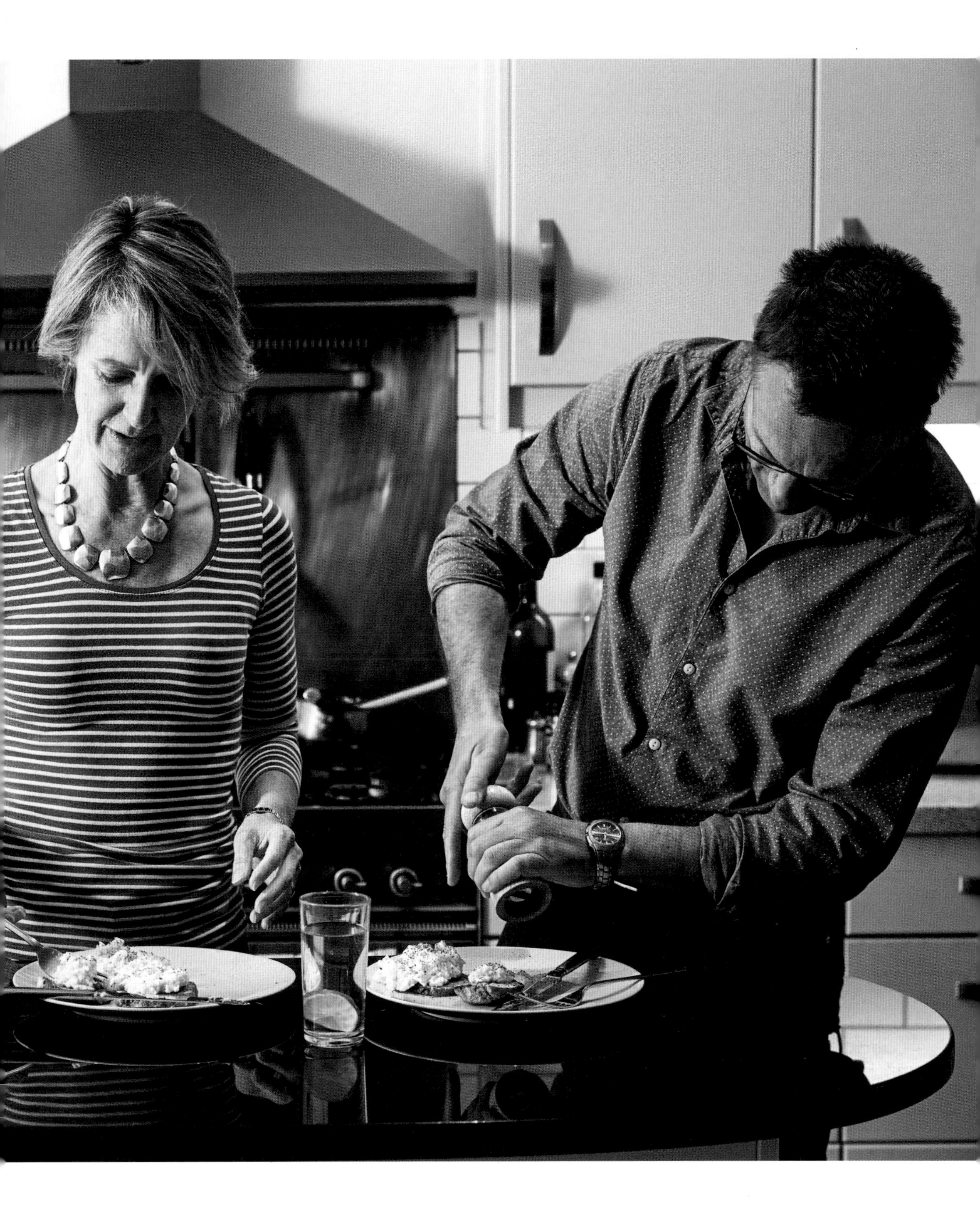

About the 8-Week Blood Sugar Diet

The 8-Week Blood Sugar Diet is based on a Mediterranean style of eating – one which is low in starchy, easily digestible carbs, but packed full of disease-fighting vitamins and flavonoids. Numerous trials have shown that not only do people get multiple health benefits from this diet, but they are also good at sticking to it (unlike those who go on a low-fat diet) because they find it easy and enjoyable. Although it is derived from the eating habits of people living in Mediterranean countries, you can apply the principles of Med-style eating to a wide range of cuisines, from Chinese or Indian through to Mexican or Scandinavian, as we have done in this book.

7 principles for low-carb Mediterranean-style eating

1. **Minimise or avoid the 'white stuff'**. The main culprits are bread, pasta, potatoes, processed cereals and rice – all refined and starchy carbohydrates which rapidly turn into sugars in the blood. Switch instead to quinoa, wholegrains, beans and lentils as these are good and filling too. Avoid just going brown: brown rice is OK, but some wholemeal breads contain added sugar, and the extra fibre added usually only has a small impact on reducing the carbohydrate load.

2. **Cut right down on sugar, sugary treats, drinks and desserts.** We offer plenty of recipes for healthy alternatives. The aim is to wean yourself off sugar.

3. **Eat more veg.** In fact, eat a rainbow, from purple beetroot through red and yellow peppers to dark leafy greens... Non-starchy vegetables are also a great way to top up on all those vital phytonutrients. We include lots of tips and simple recipes to make your vegetables irresistibly

delicious in the hope that this will encourage even the more reluctant veg eaters to increase their intake so that veg makes up half of every plate.

4. **Include some fruit, but ideally not more than 1-2 portions daily.** Go for berries, apples and pears – unpeeled, as this is where most of the nutrients are. And avoid or minimise your intake of high-sugar 'tropical' fruits such as mango, pineapple, melon and bananas.

5. **Include plenty of high-quality protein (at least 40-50g per day).** The body doesn't store protein, so you need to maintain an adequate level in your diet to avoid muscle loss. It also helps to reduce appetite. Processed meats (e.g. bacon, salami, sausages) should be eaten in moderation. High-quality proteins include meat, oily fish, eggs, seafood, tofu, soya, and, to a lesser extent nuts, chickpeas, quinoa, lentils.

6. **Enjoy your dairy products and eat more healthy fats and oils.** Until recently full-fat dairy products were shunned because of a misguided fear that they are bad for you. In 2014 a systematic review by the British Heart Foundation* which looked at the results of nearly 80 studies involving more than half a million people found no evidence that eating saturated fats leads to a greater risk of heart disease. In fact, they found that people with higher levels in their blood of a particular saturated fat called margaric acid (the sort you get in milk and dairy products) had a lower risk of heart disease. These days I encourage people to consume more fats such as olive oil, yoghurt, cheese, nuts, prawns, avocados and coconut milk. They make food taste better. They are an excellent source of slow-burn energy. And, although gram for gram they are higher in calories than carbs, they keep you full for longer. Adding fat to starchy food (butter to potatoes, for example), will actually slow the rate at which the starch is broken down into sugars and absorbed. Eating healthy oils also improves the absorption of the essential fat-soluble vitamins (A, D, E and K).

7. **Bring on the vinegar!** Vinegar has been found to help reduce weight and visceral (abdominal) fat, improve lipids and insulin sensitivity, so not surprisingly it features in a number of recipes in this book. In a recent study,** scientists found that adding 2 teaspoons of vinegar to a meal cut the post-meal blood sugar spike by 20%, while subjects in another study,*** who were asked to consume a tablespoon of vinegar a day for 12 weeks, lost 1.2kg more than those taking a placebo drink. Vinegar has been shown to suppress appetite and it also delays the breakdown of food into sugars in your gut.

---

* Association of dietary, circulating and supplement fatty acids with coronary risk http://annals.org/article.aspx?articleid=1846638)

** http://www.ncbi.nlm.nih.gov/pubmed/20068289

*** http://www.ncbi.nlm.nih.gov/pubmed/19661687

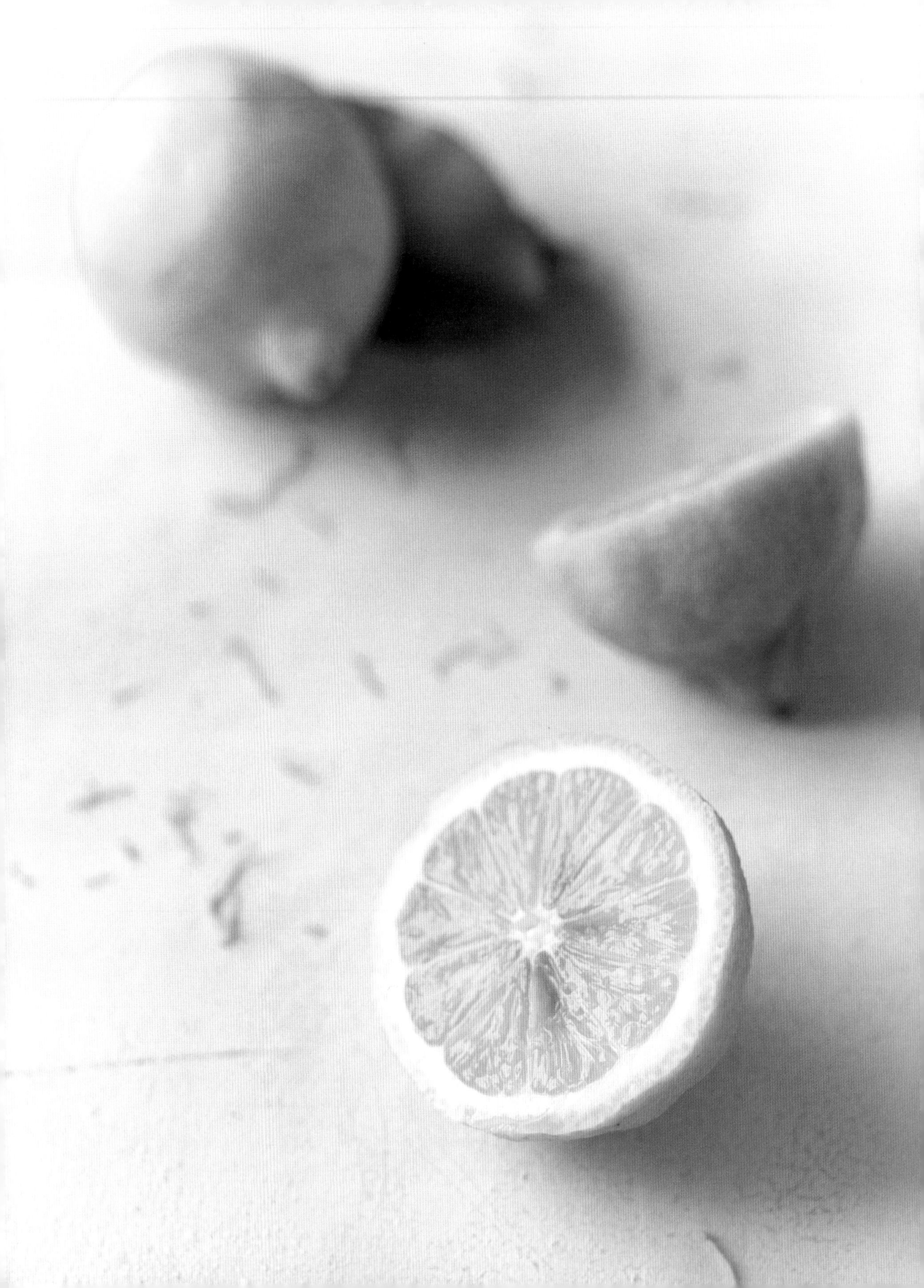

Some common questions

What are GI and GL?

Glycaemic Index (GI) is a measure of the rate at which the food you eat causes your blood sugars to rise. Low-GI foods cause blood sugar levels to rise more slowly than high-GI foods, and this helps you to feel fuller for longer. Refined and starchy carbohydrates normally have a high GI; this means they cause a spike in blood sugar levels, which then crash, leaving you feeling hungry again and so encouraging you to eat more.

The size of the spike in blood sugars is not just a result of the type of food you eat, but the amount – which is measured in Glycaemic Load (GL). Eating a big bowl of pasta is going to produce a larger, more sustained spike than eating a small bowl. For more information, go to: http://www.glycemicindex.com/

As a rule of thumb, be wary of carbs with a GI over 50, or a GL over 20, such as pasta, bread and processed cereals. Switching to lower GL versions of these staples can produce impressive improvements in blood sugar control. You should also be aware that GI and GL only relate to carbs. You won't find foods rich in protein or fat (such as chicken or butter) listed in the database above as they don't significantly affect blood sugar levels.

Can I use sweeteners?

Ideally not. We have tried to avoid use of sweeteners of any kind in our recipes, because they tend to perpetuate hunger signals and sugar cravings. Part of the aim is to help people lose their sweet tooth. So for the occasional sweet treat we aim to use sugar from fruit such as dates or include a token amount of maple syrup.

Which fats should I cook with?

Olive oil and rapeseed oil are rich in 'monounsaturated fats', which are also found in avocados, olives, almonds and hazelnuts. Monounsaturated fats are not only good for you when they are cold, they are also better at resisting damage caused by heating than the polyunsaturated fats found in sunflower and other vegetable oils. When fats and oils are heated to 'smoke point' (when frying or baking) they undergo oxidation: they react with oxygen in the air to form aldehydes and lipid peroxides. Consuming or inhaling these, even in small amounts, has been linked to increased risk of cancer and heart disease. We have chosen olive, rapeseed and coconut oils for this book as they release less of these nasty aldehydes.

We like coconut oil in particular because of its flavour, but also because there's evidence it can be helpful in reducing central obesity (i.e. visceral fat). In one study,* 40 female volunteers were randomly allocated to either 30ml of coconut oil or 30ml of soybean oil per day for 12 weeks. Unlike those consuming soybean oil, the women consuming coconut oil saw significant reductions in waist size and improvements in their cholesterol profile. For drizzling on salads and over vegetables, you might prefer the stronger, slightly nutty flavour of extra-virgin olive oil. Continue to avoid foods containing trans fats (present in many processed foods and some margarines).

Can I snack?

We recommend you keep snacking to a minimum. In the time between meals your body has a chance to go into fat-burning and repair mode. That said, we understand many people starting this diet have had fairly haphazard eating patterns as a result of busy lives and may have ended up relying on starchy meals and snacks. To counter this, we include lots of options for practical and healthy light meals or snacks to keep the wolf from the door.

How can I stay motivated?

If you are clear about why you are doing this diet, and what you want to get out of it, you will find sticking to it much easier. Consider your GOAL:

Get – what do you want to get out of it? What target do you want to get to? Is your main aim to reach a specific weight? If so, write it down. Is it to improve raised blood sugars? What level are you aiming for? To reverse diabetes? To avoid starting extra medication or starting insulin? And what is motivating you to get there?

Opportunities – what resources or opportunities do you have around you? Family? Friends? Professionals? Diet buddy? You could join the community at www.thebloodsugardiet.com

Approach – how will you approach this? What do you need to do before you start? Set up a diet diary first?

Look for successes – little by little, you should find this new approach will improve your life in all sorts of unforeseen ways. Notice the positive changes along the way and celebrate them – whether it is improved blood sugars, blood pressure or blood lipids, losing weight, or simply having more energy and feeling better. Enjoy the change.

---

* http://www.ncbi.nlm.nih.gov/pubmed/19437058

Who should *not* follow a low-calorie diet?

You should avoid a low-calorie/fasting diet if you are: underweight and/or have a history of an eating disorder, are under 18 years of age, are pregnant or breastfeeding, have a significant psychiatric disorder or are recovering from surgery. It is unwise to diet if you are unwell, frail or have a fever, or if you are under active investigation or treatment or have a significant medical condition. You should consult your doctor before starting any diet, particularly if you are on certain medications such as warfarin, insulin or drugs for diabetes or blood pressure. Likewise if you are a type 1 diabetic.

It can be helpful to confirm with your doctor that you really are a type 2 diabetic as there are other rarer forms of diabetes that will not respond in the same way to weight loss. A gentler approach may be more suitable – simply following a low-carb, Med-style approach, in which you watch your portions but don't count the calories. You can use these recipes as a guide to do that, doubling quantities and adding extra vegetables and non-starchy foods. Although it takes longer, many people get on really well with this approach.

How do I work with my health professionals?

Many doctors and health professionals are already enthusiastically on board and supporting patients doing the Blood Sugar Diet, with considerable success. Some are even doing it themselves. However, there are also health professionals who are understandably cautious about supporting new diets with which they are unfamiliar.

It may help to print the following document from Professor Roy Taylor who has helped many patients to successfully reverse their diabetes on an 800-calorie a day diet. He is a world-renowned diabetologist and has produced lots of research demonstrating the health benefits of the diet. The leaflet explains the approach and advises about medication and diabetes complications. Go to http://www.ncl.ac.uk/magres/research/diabetes/documents/Informationfordoctors_revised_April14.pdf

Either way, before you start, if you have not had your blood tested for diabetes and raised blood lipids, or your blood pressure, weight and waist measured recently, it would be worth doing so, especially if you think you might be at risk of developing diabetes. There are some helpful tests for assessing your diabetes risk on our website thebloodsugardiet.com.

N.B. The calorie count and nutritional information for each recipe is calculated per portion.

Getting started

First things first – a bit of kitchen hygiene. This doesn't mean getting the bleach out. It means removing those temptations hidden in the corners of your kitchen drawers – chocolate, biscuits, tins of rice pudding, Nutella... whatever it is that might test your resolve.

Blood Sugar Diet store cupboard essentials

If you do quite a bit of cooking, you probably already have a lot of the things in the list below. However, if you are relatively new to cooking or you are going to radically change your diet and way of eating with this recipe book, you may find it useful to go through your kitchen cupboards and then do a big stock-up at the local supermarket. You certainly don't need to buy everything on the list. But you are more likely to cook something if you have most of what you need in store.

Some of these ingredients may look unfamiliar and some frighteningly wholesome, but bear with us and try them if you can, as variety is hugely important to your diet and we are hoping to introduce you to an enjoyable and healthier way of eating. Some of the ingredients were new to us too. We are still having fun working out interesting and tasty things to make with chia seeds. (We have marked with asterixes the items that we use a lot.)

Spices

cayenne pepper
chilli flakes*
Chinese 5-spice
cinnamon (ground or sticks)
paprika*
Maldon salt*
mixed spice
nutmeg
piri piri flavouring
Saxa table salt*

Herbs

bay leaves (fresh or dried)
cardamom pods*
chilli (powder and flakes)
coriander (ground)
cumin (ground & seeds)*
curry powder (or paste)
garam masala
oregano*
tarragon
thyme*
turmeric (ground)

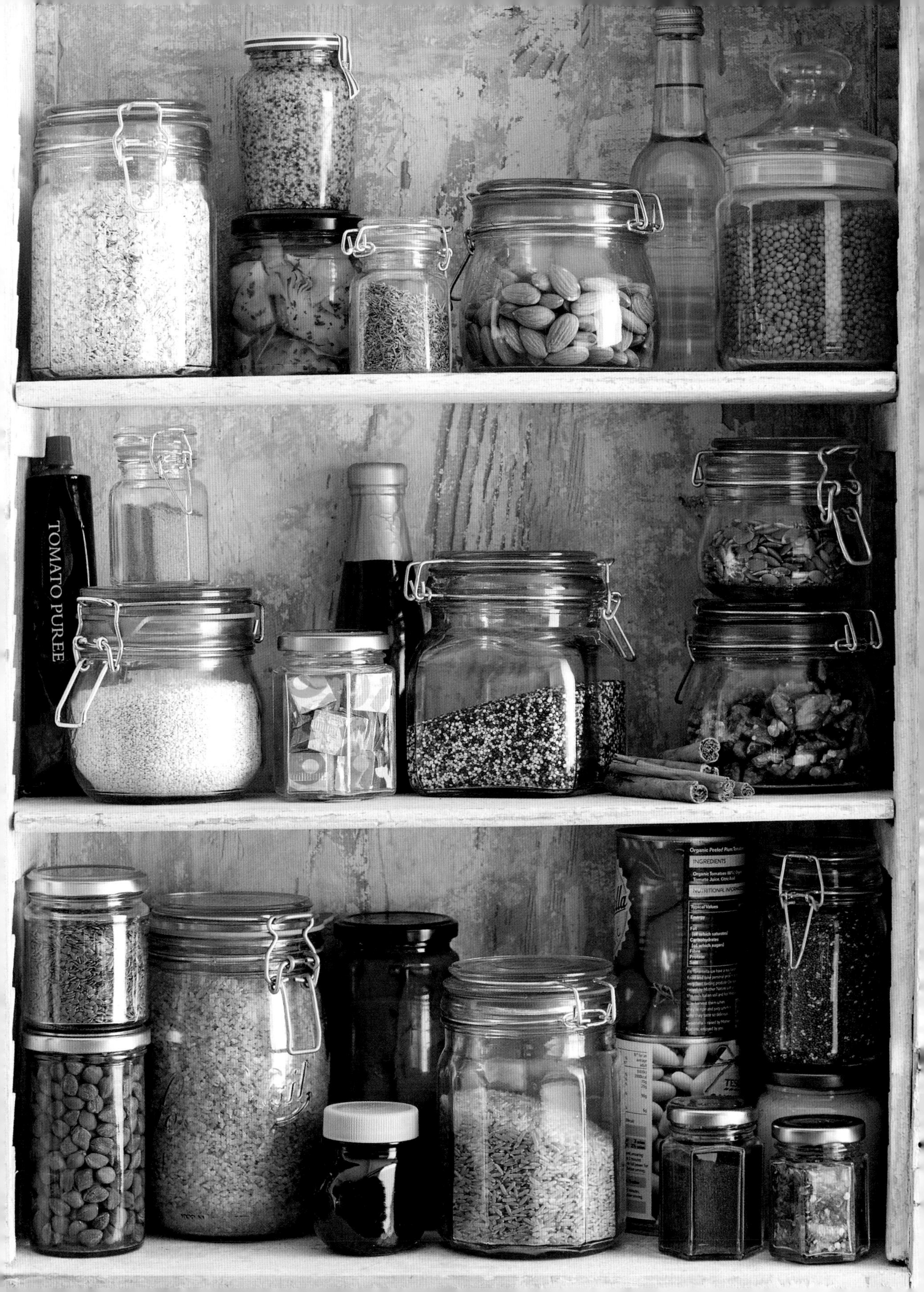
TOMATO PUREE
Organic Peeled
INGREDIENTS
Typical Values
Energy
Fat
Carbohydrates
Fibre
Protein

Grains, beans and pulses

baked beans (low-sugar)
black beans (tinned)
borlotti beans (tinned)*
brown rice*
bulgar wheat*
butterbeans (tinned or dried)
cannellini beans (tinned or dried)*
chickpeas (tinned or dried)*
kidney beans (tinned)*
lentils: black, red or green (tinned, dried or in packets)
oats (whole and rolled)*
quinoa*

Nuts and seeds

almonds (whole, flaked and/or ground)*
Brazil nuts
cashew nuts*
chia seeds*
hazelnuts
linseeds
pecans
pine nuts*
pumpkin seeds
raisins
sesame seeds
walnuts

Oils and vinegars

balsamic vinegar*
cider vinegar*
coconut oil*
extra-virgin olive oil*
olive oil*
rapeseed oil
sesame oil

Flours and baking

almond flour
baking powder*
cocoa powder
cornflour
gram flour
ground almonds*
wholemeal flour
wholemeal spelt*
wholemeal rye

Mustards, sauces and pastes

basil pesto
chilli paste
chutney or pickle
coconut cream
coconut milk (full-fat)*
harissa paste
hoisin sauce
honey
ginger paste
ginger (in syrup)
maple syrup
mayonnaise (full-fat)
mirin (Japanese rice wine)
miso paste
mustard (Dijon and wholegrain)*
soy sauce (preferably low-salt)*
stock cubes (chicken, vegetable)*
sweet chilli sauce
Tabasco
Thai fish sauce*
tomato purée*
Worcestershire sauce

Tinned fish

anchovies*
sardines*
tuna*

Vegetables and fruit in tins or jars

artichoke hearts
beansprouts
black or green olives*
capers
grapefruit
lychees
roasted red peppers
sushi pickled ginger (optional)
tomatoes*

Jams and spreads

cashew or almond nut butter
Marmite

In the freezer

chicken breasts (individually wrapped)
cooked brown rice, quinoa, bulgar wheat (in portions) edamame beans
fish (salmon fillet, cod or other white fish)
fruits (berries, rhubarb, plums)
peas*
prawns*
spinach*

Dried fruit

soft apricots
soft dates*

In the fridge

berries (raspberries, blueberries, strawberries*)
cheese (Parmesan, strong Cheddar, feta, halloumi)
chillies*
crème fraîche
free-range eggs
full-fat Greek yoghurt
garlic*
lemons and limes
non-starchy vegetables (cauliflower, broccoli, courgette, cherry tomatoes, cucumber, peppers, radishes, lettuce, greens)
root ginger*

Useful equipment

non-stick saucepans
non-stick frying pan and wok
non-stick omelette pan
cast-iron casserole dish suitable for hobs as well as ovens
ramekins for baking small portions
short wooden sticks (for kebabs)
potato masher
lemon squeezer
spiraliser (see page 107)
large and small measuring jugs
food processor or hand blender

12 TIPS for 800-cal fasting days

1. Plan in advance and aim for variety to maintain interest and nutritional balance. Many people have meals planned, or even ready the day before, so they don't give into temptation. We suggest ideas for quick and easy dishes to assemble the night before so you can dash out in the morning with a healthy breakfast on board, as well as tips for preparing something that you can have ready and waiting for you when you get home from work.

   The first 2 weeks might be tough, but most people find their body gets used to it. As their stomach shrinks and their insulin resistance improves, most people find their constant cravings settle and they don't want so much to eat. In fact, the majority of people say that they feel hugely better and have more energy.

2. Increase water intake to reduce the side effects of calorie cutting, such as tiredness, lightheadedness and headaches (these are often related to dehydration and sometimes insufficient salt intake), hunger (this comes in waves and passes so try to 'surf the wave') and feeling colder. Aim for 2-3 litres a day. You can also add a bit more salt to food or use Marmite/ Vegemite.

3. Drink soup as it's surprisingly satiating as well as cheap and practical. You can take it to work for lunch and keep portions in the freezer.

4. Use low-carb alternatives for potatoes, pasta, rice. We have included all sorts of tips and tricks to help you with this. Try grated cauliflower instead of rice, spiralised vegetables or finely sliced cabbage instead of pasta or noodles.

5. Avoid sugar and sweet syrups wherever possible, even if they are 'natural' sugars. Where a savoury dish needs a touch of sweetness use whole fruit if you can; its impact is reduced when it is eaten with fats and fibre, which slows its absorption.

6. Drink hot drinks to suppress your appetite: teas, coffee, Bovril, miso soup etc.

7. Beware hidden calories in drinks. Alcohol is surprisingly high-calorie so avoid it if possible during the diet. Other unexpected liquid calories include fruit juice, smoothies and cordials.

8. Avoid 'diet' products as they often contain sugar and/or sweeteners to make them more palatable. And they don't reduce sweet cravings.

9. Build in strong flavours with the likes of lemon, pepper, lime, chilli, garlic, gherkins, mustard and herbs. It is a great way of making food more satisfying.

10. Use a nutritional counter such as My Fitness Pal to measure and track your meals, especially if you are not always following the menu planner in this book, to ensure that you get a healthy nutritional balance in your diet. (That said, be aware that while these calorie and food analysis tools can be very helpful, you shouldn't get too concerned about variations between them. The calorie counts are only intended as a guide and different systems may produce different results.)

11. Take multivitamins at least every other day, if you can, particularly if you are doing 800 calories for more than a few weeks. The recipes have been designed to ensure that you get a balanced diet with adequate protein, fat and nutrients but a multivitamin won't hurt.

12. Share meals with others where possible. It is important not to become isolated on any diet. Just remember to have smaller portions of the same food where you can and skip the carbs. Friends and family might benefit too…

What do I do once I have achieved my goals?

Once you have reached your target weight and/or got your blood sugars down to healthy levels, it is vital that you do not slip back into a starchy or high-sugar diet as that will eventually undo all the good work. So for maintenance we recommend the Blood Sugar Diet Way of Life.*

The recipes in this book provide an excellent basis for healthy eating and keeping weight and blood sugar down indefinitely. When you are no longer counting the calories, use the recipes as a guide, sticking to the principles of the Mediterranean way of eating, and simply increasing the quantities to roughly double, adding more non-starchy vegetables and including more wholegrain foods. Some people, when they come off the intensive diet, continue to do an 800-calorie day once or even twice a week to keep their weight and blood sugars on track.

What we hope, above all, is that you have absorbed enough about the core principles of healthy eating from this book to be able to build them into a flexible and sustainable way of life that suits you personally. That is when dieting is successful.

---

* For more advice and support we recommend you join the active and well-informed community at thebloodsugardiet.com

Breakfast and Brunch

Breakfast tends to be the most underrated meal of the day, often eaten on your feet, and made up of instant cereals or a piece of toast and jam – neither of which will keep you going. The starchy carbs are burnt quickly and send your blood sugars soaring, only to crash a few hours later to leave you bewilderingly hungry and craving a midday snack.

We predict a revolution in breakfast-eating habits over the next decade – one in which Blood Sugar dieters will be ahead of the game. Prepare to banish those dreary old processed cereals for good. Start the day instead with an energy-boosting combination of protein and plants: eggs, avocados, fish, tomatoes, mushrooms, spinach… we guarantee you will never look back.

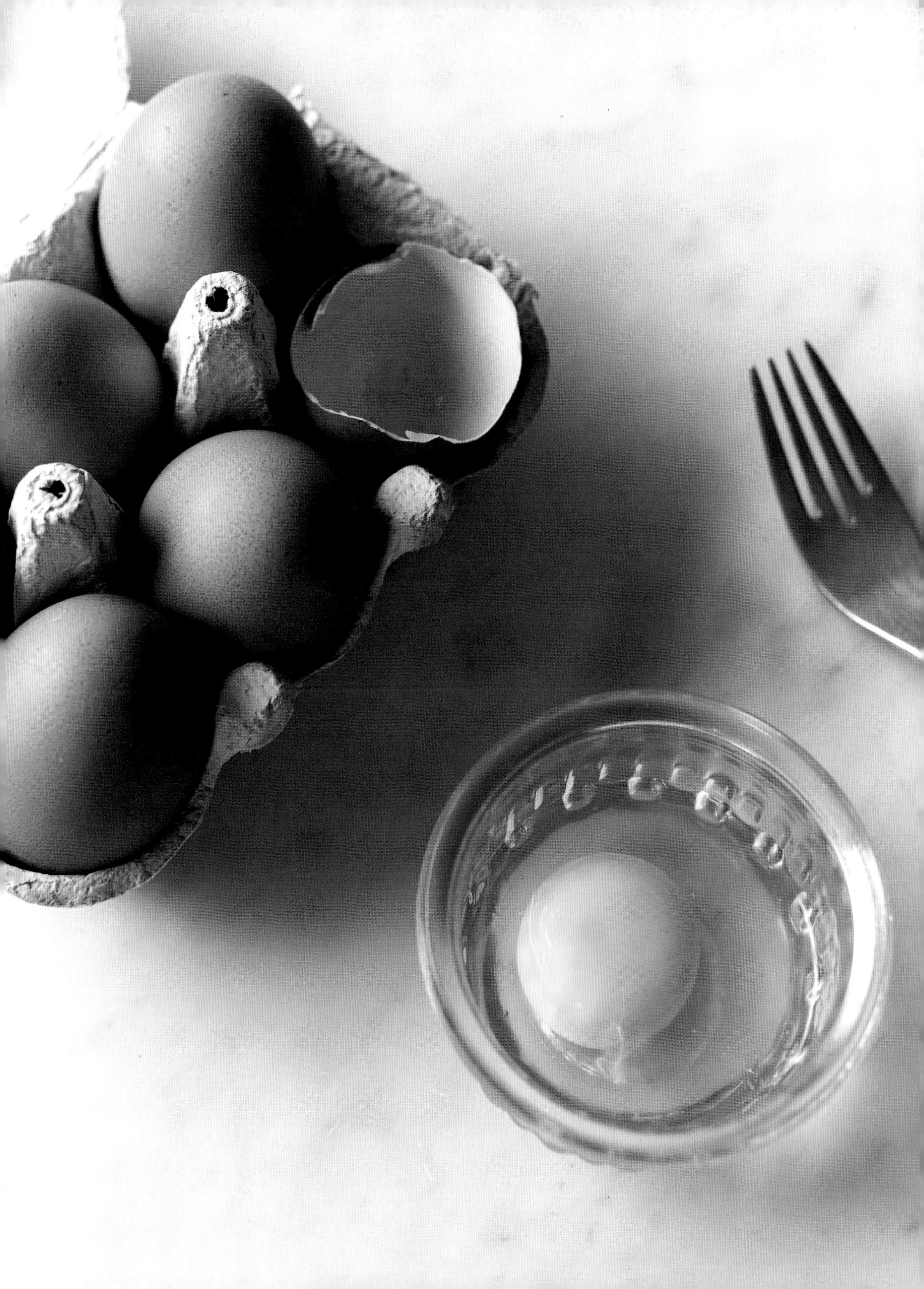

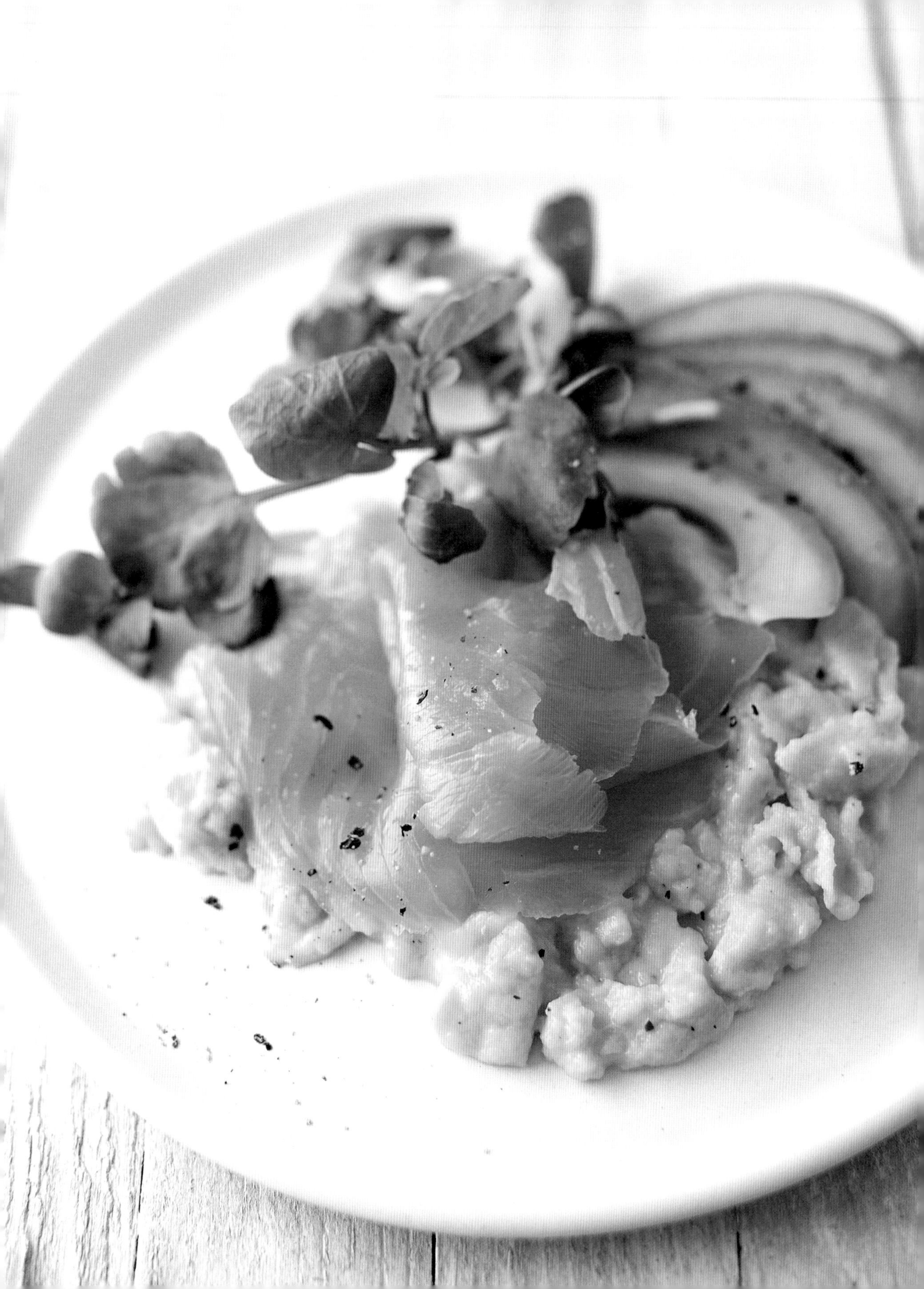

Quick, easy breakfasts

Michael's perfect scrambled eggs

Serves 1

2 eggs
Small knob of butter (or dash of oil)

Whisk the eggs in a cup or bowl with a fork. In a small non-stick pan, heat the butter gently until it melts (don't allow it to brown), then add the eggs. Stir slowly and continuously with a wooden spoon or spatula for 1-2 minutes to produce a creamy consistency. Remove from the heat while it is still runny in places as it will go on cooking in the pan.

- CALORIES 200
- PROTEIN 13G
- FAT 17G
- FIBRE 0G
- CARBS 0G

Try some of the variations below, all made with 2 medium eggs:

With chilli: add flavour with a scattering of dried chilli or fresh chives.

With smoked salmon: (add 90 cals) this is Michael's routine breakfast. Scramble 2 eggs, and serve with 50g chopped smoked salmon and freshly ground black pepper. You can also add ¼ medium avocado, sliced (add 60 cals).

With fried mushrooms: (add 20 cals) mushrooms are low in carbs, high in protein and fibre and amazingly filling given their low calorie count. They also contain high levels of vitamin D. Fry 80g mushrooms in a non-stick pan with a drizzle of oil until golden brown (4-5 minutes). Meanwhile, prepare the scrambled eggs. Assemble together on a plate and season with salt and black pepper.

Green eggs and ham: (add 50 cals) this is an excellent way to use up leftover greens from the night before. Simply stir in a handful, or some fresh spinach. Serve with a couple of slices of ham 40-50g.

Why we love eggs

Eggs are nutrient-dense, vitamin-rich, high in protein and healthy fatty acids, naturally vacuum-wrapped, fast to cook and incredibly flexible. They also keep you full for longer, without pushing up your blood sugars or cholesterol. Yes! Many of my patients are surprised to hear me recommending eggs, a legacy of the years in which they were unfairly blamed for raising blood cholesterol levels. Let me reassure you: eggs are fine.

Simple omelette

Delicious on its own or with tasty extras thrown in.

Serves 1

2 eggs
Small knob of butter (or a dash of oil)

Gently whisk the eggs with a fork in a cup or bowl. Add pepper and salt to taste. In a small non-stick frying pan, heat the butter and spread it around the pan until it bubbles, then pour in the eggs. After a few seconds lower the heat and cook it until the underside is golden brown. Fold the omelette in two and serve it while it's still a bit runny on the surface (it will go on cooking on the plate). Perfect.

- **CALORIES** 200
- PROTEIN 13G
- FAT 17G
- FIBRE 0G
- CARBS 0G

Mushroom omelette

Serves 1

80g mushrooms, sliced
2 eggs
Small knob of butter (or a dash of oil)

Sauté the mushrooms in a drizzle of oil until they are golden brown (4-5 minutes). Gently whisk the eggs with a fork in a cup or bowl. Add salt and pepper to taste. For the omelette, heat the butter in a small non-stick frying pan, and spread it around the pan until it bubbles, then pour in the eggs. After a few seconds lower the heat, add the cooked mushrooms and cook the omelette until the underside is golden brown. Fold it in two and serve it while it is still a bit runny on the surface (it will go on cooking on the plate).

- **CALORIES** 210
- PROTEIN 14G
- FAT 17G
- FIBRE 1G
- CARBS 0G

Poached eggs with spinach and pine nuts

Serves 1

1 tsp wine or cider vinegar
2 eggs
1 tsp butter
200g spinach
¼ tsp ground nutmeg
1 tsp pine nuts, toasted
10g (1 tbsp) Parmesan, grated

Bring a pan of water to the boil, add the vinegar and reduce the heat to a simmer. Crack the eggs into the water and poach them for 3 minutes. Melt the butter in a pan and add the spinach. Sprinkle on the nutmeg, a pinch of salt and plenty of black pepper and allow the spinach to wilt over a gentle heat. Drain it in a colander and place it on a plate, topped with the eggs and a sprinkle of Parmesan cheese and pine nuts.

- **CALORIES** 290
- PROTEIN 17G
- FAT 24G
- FIBRE 1G
- CARBS 1G

Kipper and tomatoes

Another easy, healthy default breakfast. Kippers are good value and full of wonderful fish oils. They are very practical too as they keep for a few days in the fridge or can be frozen. The ones in a packet take 2-3 minutes in a microwave – about as long as it takes to make a cup of tea. For extra oomph, sprinkle them with chilli flakes and freshly ground black pepper.

Serves 1

1 smoked kipper (or mackerel fillet)
Knob of butter
100g tomatoes

Grill or microwave the smoked fish with a knob of butter according to instructions. Serve it on a bed of tomatoes, either cold or cooked (see overnight tomatoes, page 39).

Tip: on a non-fasting day, serve it with a small piece of seeded spelt and rye toast (see bread options on pages 180-81).

- **CALORIES** 230
- PROTEIN 10G
- FAT 20G
- FIBRE 1G
- CARBS 3G

Big mushrooms with feta

These are also known as Portobello mushrooms. We received an email recently from a gentleman who said he was inclined to give up on recipes with words such as falafel, frittata, harissa, Portobello, julienne strips… and fair enough. For this book, we have tried to keep the names of ingredients as simple and unpretentious as possible. So 'Big mushrooms' it is… cooked with feta and olive oil. Delicious they are too.

Serves 1

60g spinach, roughly chopped
30g feta, crumbled
Pinch of ground nutmeg
2-3 large flat mushrooms
1 tbsp olive oil

Preheat the oven to 180°C. Wilt the spinach in a pan, drain it well and squeeze out excess water. Place it in a bowl and stir in the feta with some salt and pepper and the nutmeg.

Remove the stalks from the mushrooms, and brush them all over with olive oil. Place them on a baking tray flat side down and fill them with the spinach mixture. Bake them for 15 minutes.

- **CALORIES** 180
- PROTEIN 7G
- FAT 10G
- FIBRE 2G
- CARBS 2G

Avocados with pre-baked tomatoes

Avocados are brimming with essential nutrients, including potassium, B vitamins and folic acid. They also contain large amounts of the healthy monounsaturated fat, oleic acid, and have at last been acknowledged as having beneficial, health-promoting properties similar to those of olive oil.

Serves 2

200g tomatoes (about 3 medium-sized)
½ tsp dried tarragon, oregano or rosemary
2 ripe avocados
½ tsp paprika
Pinch of chilli flakes (optional)

Cut the tomatoes in half, scatter with the herbs and bake them in the oven for 30 minutes (or use pre-baked tomatoes, see page 39). Cut the avocados in half, scoop out the flesh and divide it between two plates. Then mash it roughly, top it with the tomatoes and serve it with the paprika, chilli and black pepper sprinkled over.

- **CALORIES** 300
- PROTEIN 4G
- FAT 29G
- FIBRE 7G
- CARBS 8G

Avocado and feta bash

Serves 2

1 ripe avocado
Handful of parsley or basil, chopped.
1 tbsp olive oil
1 tbsp walnuts, toasted or hazelnuts for crunch
30g feta, crumbled
¼ tsp chilli flakes

Cut the avocado in half and scoop the flesh out into a bowl. Mash it with the herbs, olive oil, nuts, feta and chilli along with some seasoning. Divide the mixture between 2 plates.

Tip: if you are on a non-fasting day you could serve it on a small piece of seeded spelt and rye bread (see page 181), toasted and lightly rubbed with garlic.

- **CALORIES** 460
- PROTEIN 9G
- FAT 46G
- FIBRE 5G
- CARBS 3G

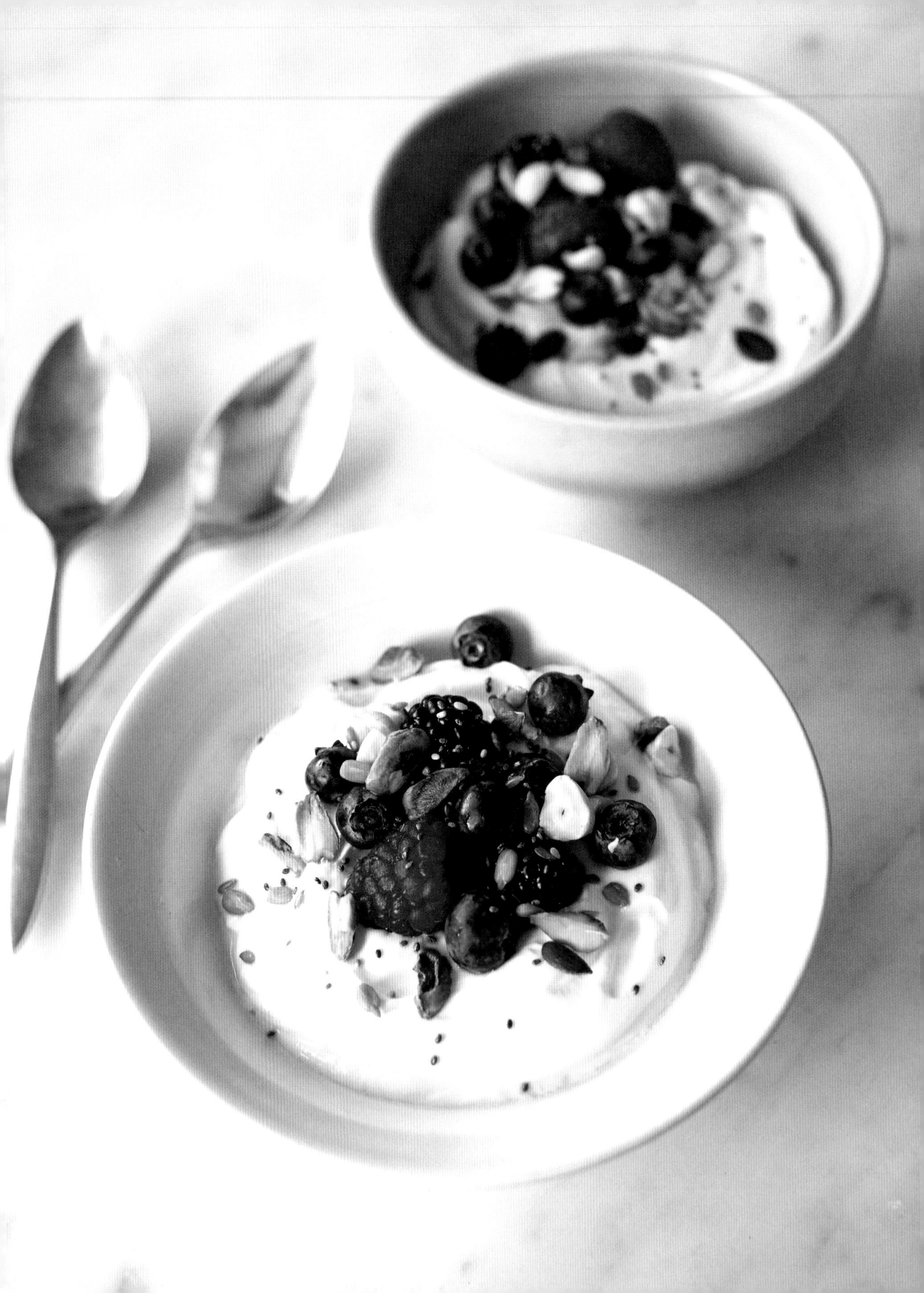

In praise of full-fat Greek yoghurt

Full-fat dairy products are a staple part of the Mediterranean diet, and have now thankfully been reinstated on the official good food list in the UK, after a long time out in the cold. We generally recommend Greek-style yoghurt as it has been strained to retain a higher protein content. It is satiating without significantly raising blood sugar and there is now clear evidence that a diet containing dairy products does not cause diabetes or have an undue impact on cholesterol.

Live, unsweetened yoghurt will also help boost the healthy bacteria in your gut. The trouble with low-fat yoghurts is that they tend to contain a lot of added sugar or sweeteners and starchy thickeners which kill these vital bacteria. So beware.

We have recently discovered full-fat coconut yoghurt as a delicious non-dairy alternative: it has a naturally sweet taste, is dairy-free and contains healthy fat and minimal starchy carbohydrate. It is more expensive than normal yoghurt, but otherwise fits the bill.

Greek yoghurt with nuts, seeds and berries

Toasting nuts and seeds transforms their taste – the heat sets off a chemical reaction which enhances the flavour.

Serves 1

2 large tbsp Greek yoghurt
1 tbsp (15g) toasted seeds or nuts of your choice (sunflower seeds, pumpkin seeds, almonds, hazelnuts, walnuts)
Small handful of berries (raspberries, strawberries, blackberries or blueberries, according to what is in season)

Assemble in a bowl and tuck in.

- **CALORIES** 200
- PROTEIN 9G
- FAT 18G
- FIBRE 2G
- CARBS 5G

5 ways with porridge

All calories are not equal, and nor are all oats. Depending on how refined or processed the oats are, there is a significant difference in impact on blood sugars. At the healthiest end of the scale is coarse oatmeal, made of relatively unrefined steel-cut (pinhead) oats, also known as Irish oats, which retain the nutritious inner kernel, are more chewy and require soaking and cooking for up to an hour. They have a lower GI and a slower release, keeping you fuller for longer. They contain lots of fibre, of both the soluble and insoluble kind, which contributes to keeping blood sugars down and supporting healthy gut bacteria.

Unfortunately, many people are eating 'instant' porridge in the belief that it is good for them. Processed quick oats have less fibre and a high GI: they contain a more refined form of carbohydrate, which results in a significantly greater impact on blood sugars due to the carbohydrate being digested and released faster into the blood, making you feel hungry again, sooner.

Somewhere in between sit the jumbo oats and the slightly more processed rolled oats which are commonly used for breakfast porridge. We have mainly included recipes with rolled oats here, for the sake of speed and on the basis that these are certainly better for you than most breakfast cereals. But if you can, try and make sure that you have the chewy, less processed variety of oat. It takes longer to cook, but is worth it.

1. Apple and cinnamon porridge

Cinnamon reduces the speed at which the stomach empties and has been shown to lower blood sugar. It also has natural sweetness which helps reduce sugar intake.

Serves 1

25g rolled oats
175ml semi-skimmed milk
1 apple, grated
½ tsp ground cinnamon

Put the oats and milk in a saucepan, along with the grated apple and cinnamon. Add a pinch of salt to enhance the flavours. Bring it to the boil and then simmer gently for about 5 minutes, stirring frequently so it doesn't stick to the bottom of the pan.

- CALORIES 260
- PROTEIN 9G
- FAT 9G
- FIBRE 4G
- CARBS 38G

2. Extra-filling porridge with nut butter

Serves 1

25g rolled oats
175ml semi-skimmed milk
½ tsp chia seeds

For the nut butter:
100g cashews (4 servings = 25g per portion)

To make the nut butter, roast the cashews on a baking sheet in the oven at 180°C for 8-10 minutes. Allow them to cool, then blitz them in a food processor until smooth. (The butter can be stored in a jar with a lid for up to 5 days.)

To make the porridge, put the oats and milk in a saucepan, along with 1 tbsp nut butter and a pinch of salt. Bring it to the boil and then simmer gently for about 5 minutes, stirring frequently so that it doesn't stick to the bottom of the pan. (You can also microwave it in a high-sided bowl, covered, for 3-4 minutes.) Scatter the chia seeds over the surface and serve.

- **CALORIES** 310
- PROTEIN 12G
- FAT 17G
- FIBRE 3G
- CARBS 28G

---

3. Medium oatmeal porridge

According to the latest research, coconut oil can help you lose weight and reduce 'dangerous' abdominal fat. It is made up of medium-chain fatty acids which are metabolised differently from the much commoner, longer-chain fats. A study of 14 healthy men found that those who ate medium-chain fatty acids such as coconut oil at breakfast ate significantly fewer calories at lunch.*

Serves 1

25g medium (pinhead) oatmeal
150ml water
75ml semi-skimmed milk
1 tsp coconut oil
½ tsp ground cinnamon or ginger
Pinch of salt
1 fig, chopped

Put the oats in a saucepan and soak them overnight in the water (enough to just cover them).

In the morning, add the milk, coconut oil and cinnamon and simmer for about 5 minutes, stirring frequently. Serve it with the fig scattered on top.

- **CALORIES** 290
- PROTEIN 10G
- FAT 15G
- FIBRE 3G
- CARBS 31G

* http://www.ncbi.nlm.nih.gov/pubmed/9701177)

4. Spicy fruit porridge

Serves 1

1 small apple or pear, skin on, cored and diced
½ tsp mixed spice
Knob of butter
25g rolled oats
175ml semi-skimmed milk

Dust the apple pieces in the mixed spice, fry them briefly with a knob of butter and set them aside. Put the oats and milk in a saucepan with a pinch of salt. Bring it to the boil, then simmer gently for about 5 minutes, stirring frequently. Serve it with the spiced apple piled on top.

- **CALORIES** 210
- PROTEIN 9G
- FAT 5G
- FIBRE 3G
- CARBS 34G

---

5. Pecan chia porridge with raspberries

Set yourself up for the day with this very pleasing variation on porridge. It has a delicate flavour which you wouldn't immediately recognise as Earl Grey and which contrasts deliciously with the berries and nuts.

Serves 2

1 Earl Grey tea bag
250ml semi-skimmed milk
1 tbsp chia seeds (20g)
25g rolled oats
175g raspberries (or strawberries or blueberries)
3 tbsp full-fat Greek yogurt
1 tbsp pecans, chopped

Steep the tea bag in 50ml boiling water for 1 minute, then stir with a teaspoon and press out excess fluid before discarding the bag.

Place the milk, chia seeds, oats, berries (reserving a few for garnish) and tea in a small saucepan and simmer gently for 2-3 minutes, stirring frequently. Leave it to cool slightly before transferring it to a bowl.

Stir in the yoghurt and cool the mixture in the fridge for 30 minutes or longer, to allow it to set a little. Top it with the remaining berries and sprinkle over the nuts.

- **CALORIES** 230
- PROTEIN 15G
- FAT 27G
- FIBRE 4G
- CARBS 15G

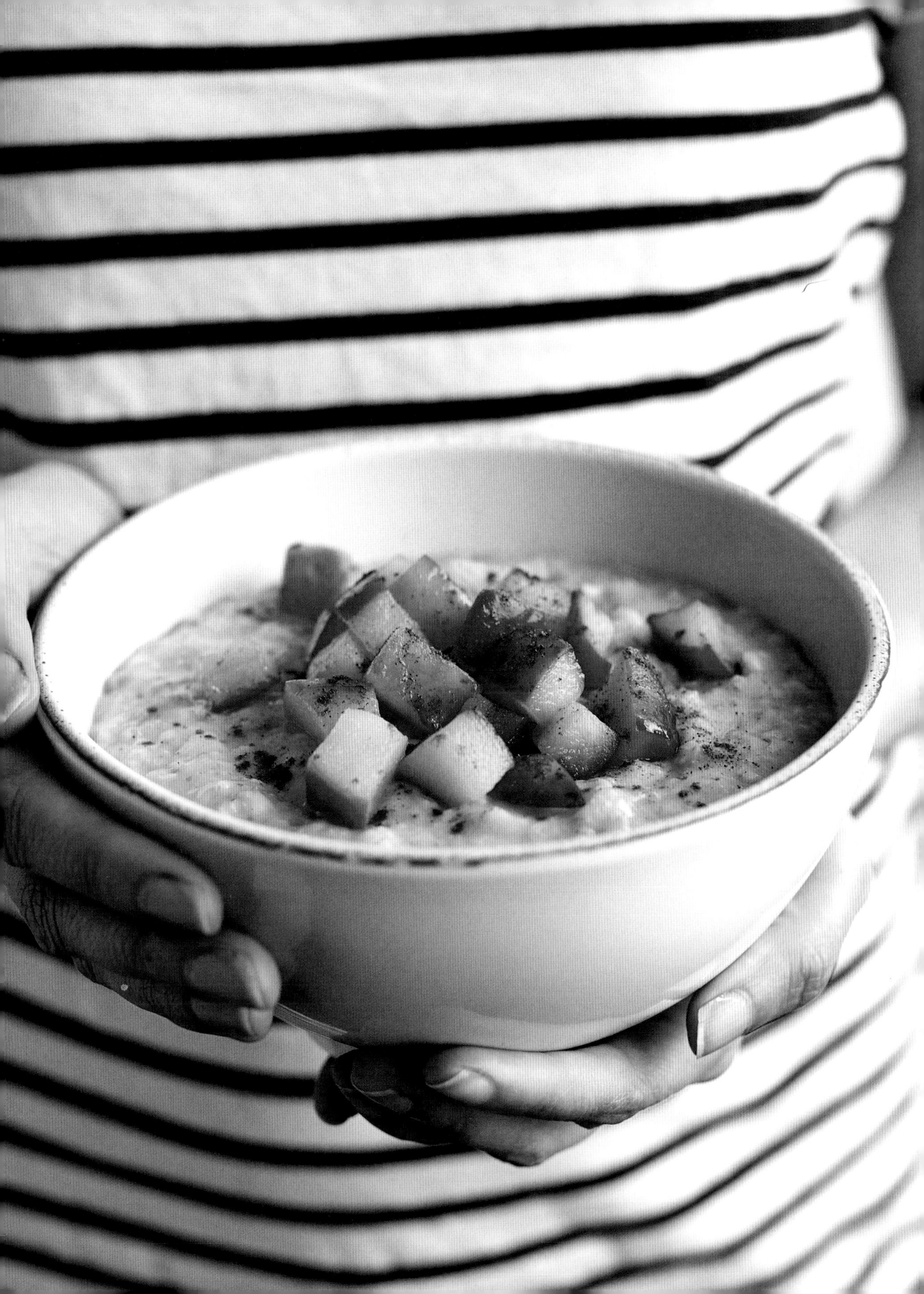

Chia breakfast bircher

Chia is amazingly high in nutrients – particularly rich in omega 3, an important fatty acid which protects the cardiovascular system and improves cholesterol. It is a relatively new discovery for us and we are enjoying its flexibility. Although it has little flavour of its own, chia can be scattered over almost any food or mixed in to create a creamy texture.

Serves 2

1 tbsp chia seeds
30g rolled porridge oats, with bran
½ 400ml tin coconut milk
2 passion fruit (or a squeeze of lemon and zest of half a lemon)
2 ripe figs, chopped (or a handful of berries)
1 tbsp hazelnuts, toasted and chopped

Combine the chia seeds, oats and coconut milk together, then divide the mixture between 2 small bowls and allow it to stand for at least 30 minutes. (It is even better prepared the night before and kept in the fridge.) Scoop out the seeds from the passion fruit and stir them into the bircher. Serve it topped with the chopped figs and nuts.

- **CALORIES** 340
- PROTEIN 6G
- FAT 27G
- FIBRE 3G
- CARBS 20G

Advance prep tips

- **Chop and put aside ingredients to add to an omelette or scrambled eggs the night before** – look out for tasty leftovers, such as a handful of meat, cheese or cooked greens.

- **Make your porridge the day before** so you can simply reheat it in the microwave with an extra tablespoon of milk, depending on your preferred consistency.

- **Roast tomatoes overnight** – perfect tomatoes, ready when you wake, adapted from a neat idea by Nigella, who cooks them slowly overnight as the oven cools.

  Serves 2
  200g (3-4) medium-sized tomatoes, halved
  1 tsp dried thyme or tarragon
  Salt, pepper and a dash of olive oil

  Preheat the oven to 200°C. Place the tomatoes cut side up on a baking dish. Scatter with the herbs, drizzle over the olive oil and season with salt and black pepper. Place the tray on the top shelf of the oven and turn the oven off. By the morning, your roasted tomatoes will be ready and waiting. Serve them with kippers or half an avocado for a fantastically healthy breakfast.

- **Keep ready-toasted seeds at hand** – nuts and seeds taste sweeter toasted, so prepare a bulk batch by either dry-frying them in a pan, or browning them under the grill or in the oven. You need to watch closely as they can burn easily. Store them in small clean jam jars with lids, ready to sprinkle on anything from yoghurt or porridge to salads.

- **Prepare hard-boiled eggs the day before** – for an instant getaway, boil two eggs for 7 minutes, then dunk them in a bowl of cold water and pat them dry. When you're ready to eat them, simply peel them and season them with salt and pepper.

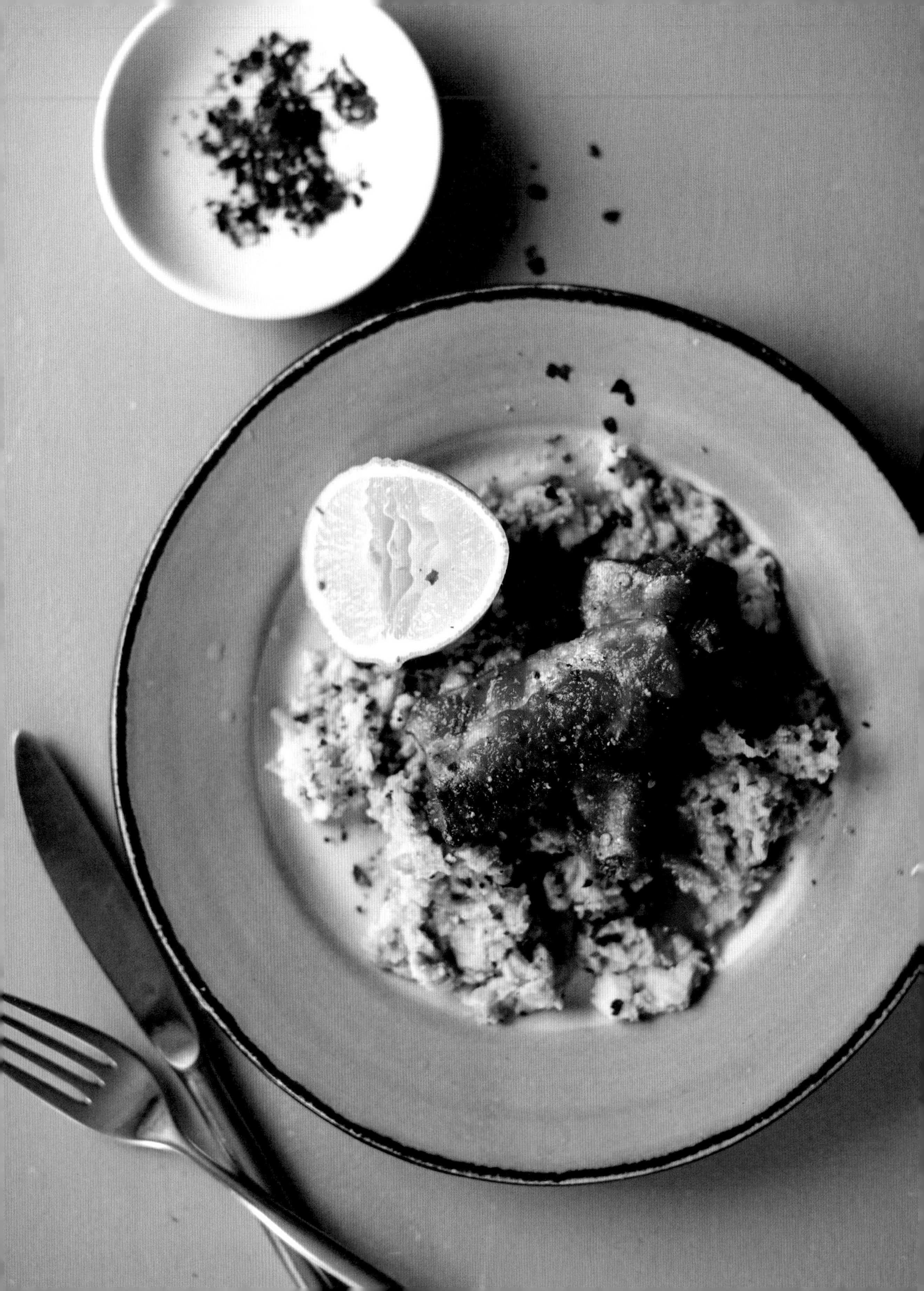

Brunch

These are more substantial dishes, perhaps best for the weekend when you get up a bit later and breakfast merges into lunch. Some take slightly longer to prepare than the quick breakfasts – but they will keep you going well into the day without a sugar spike in sight.

Sardines on avocado mash

A great combination which is incredibly filling and contains oodles of wonderful omega 3. It is also very quick to make.

Serves 1

60g (½ tin) sardines in tomato sauce
1 avocado, roughly mashed
Squeeze of lime

Lay the sardines on top of the avocado mash, squeeze over the lime juice and season with salt and freshly ground black pepper (chilli flakes too, if you like).

- CALORIES 370
- PROTEIN 13G
- FAT 34G
- FIBRE 5G
- CARBS 4G

Ham and cheese omelette

A more substantial omelette, with a crucial extra bit of protein to keep hunger at bay.

Serves 1

2 eggs
50g ham, sliced
Knob of butter (or a dash of oil)
15g Cheddar, grated

Gently whisk the eggs with a fork in a cup or bowl and add the cooked ham and salt and pepper to taste. In a small non-stick frying pan, heat the butter and spread it around the pan until it bubbles, then pour in the mixture. After a few seconds lower the heat, sprinkle the cheese on top and cook the omelette until the underside is golden brown. Fold it in half and let it cook for a bare minute more. Serve it while it's still a bit runny on the surface (it goes on cooking on the plate). Try with a scattering of chilli flakes to add flavour.

See pages 28 and 55 for more omelette recipes.

- **CALORIES** 340
- PROTEIN 26G
- FAT 26G
- FIBRE 1G
- CARBS 0G

Simple egg muffins

Adapted from a lovely recipe on the Blood Sugar Diet website by Aliba. Easy to make with everyday ingredients and delicious hot or cold, they make an excellent portable breakfast, brunch or lunch. Any extra muffins can be frozen.

Serves 6 - makes 6 muffins in a standard muffin tray

100g mushrooms, finely chopped
Small knob of butter
4 eggs
100g full-fat cottage cheese
4-5 rashers of bacon
40g Cheddar, grated, or feta, crumbled
Handful of baby spinach leaves, shredded (or a handful of pre-cooked greens)

Preheat the oven to 180°C. Fry the mushrooms in the butter in a non-stick pan, then set them aside. Beat the eggs with the cottage cheese and season. Cut the bacon to roughly the size needed to line the base of a 6-hole muffin tray. Add the mushrooms, cheese and spinach to each muffin hole, pour over the egg mixture and bake for 30-35 minutes.

- **CALORIES** 130
- PROTEIN 11G
- FAT 10G
- FIBRE 0G
- CARBS 1G

Egg baked in avocado

Serves 2

1 large avocado
Pinch of paprika
2 small eggs
1 slice of smoked salmon, chopped
¼ red chilli, deseeded and finely chopped (or ¼ tsp chilli flakes)
Squeeze of lime juice

Preheat the oven to 200ºC. Using a spoon, scoop out a third of the avocado flesh, leaving 2cm-thick walls. Place each avocado half, cut side up, in a loaf tin, to keep them upright. Sprinkle each with paprika. Crack an egg into each avocado half, and then arrange the chopped smoked salmon pieces evenly on top. Bake them for 10 minutes.

Meanwhile, mash the remaining avocado flesh in a small bowl and mix it with the chilli and lime juice and some black pepper to make a dip.

- **CALORIES** 230
- PROTEIN 10G
- FAT 20G
- FIBRE 3G
- CARBS 1G

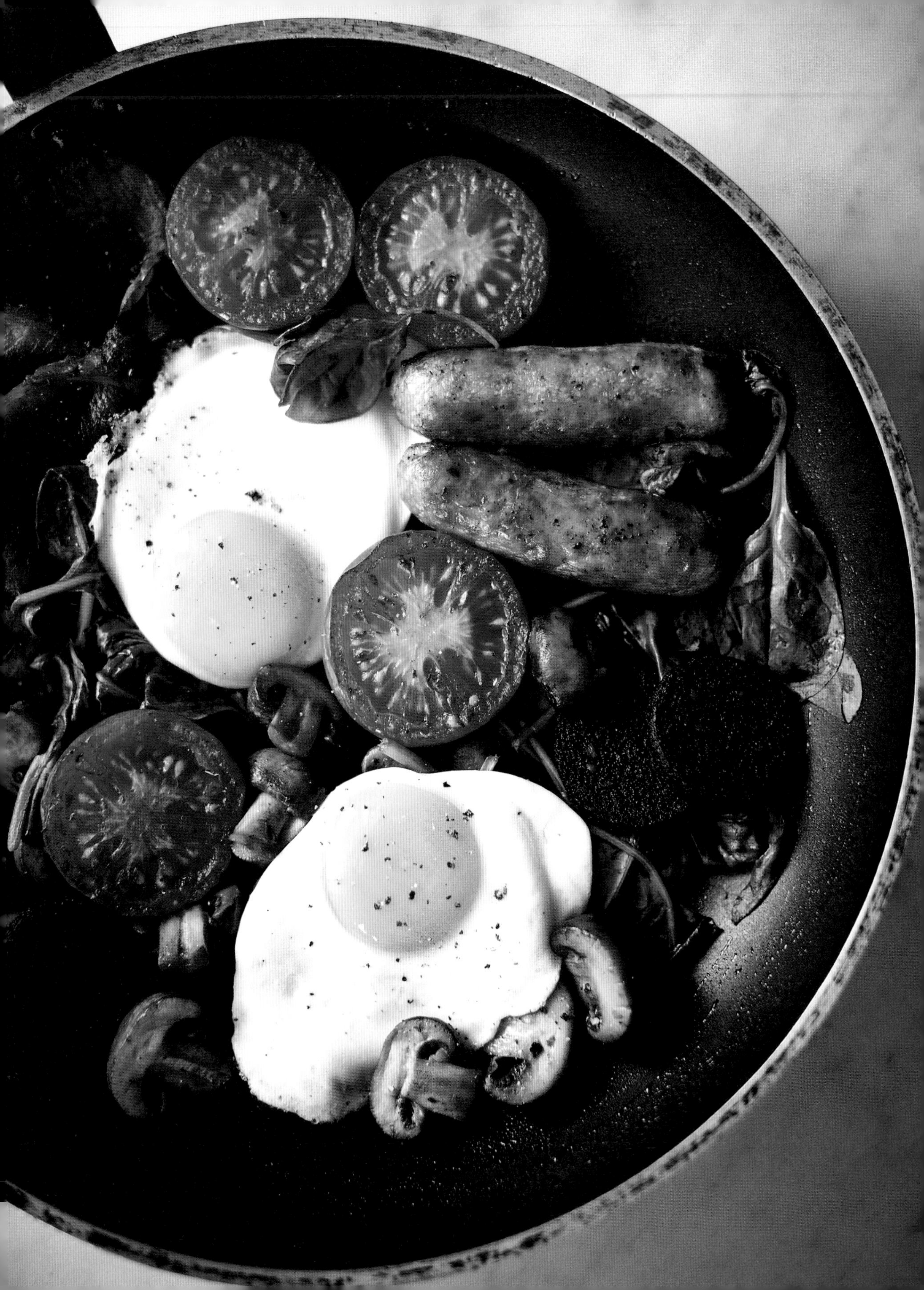

Full English breakfast

... just without the toast. This can be easily expanded for lots of people, and makes a great weekend treat.

Serves 2

2 tsp olive oil
2 rashers of free-range back bacon
2 high-meat sausages
200g mushrooms, sliced
2 large slices or 4 small slices of black pudding
2 medium-sized tomatoes, halved
2 eggs
100g spinach

Turn on the oven to 100°C to keep things warm as you cook them. Place a large frying pan over a moderate to high heat, add 1 tsp olive oil and fry the bacon and sausages. Put them in an ovenproof dish in the oven. In the same oil, fry the mushrooms, and transfer them to the dish in the oven. Next fry the tomatoes for 2-3 minutes on each side and put them in the oven too.

Now, add the other tsp oil, fry the black pudding, and finally the eggs (or scramble these in a small non-stick pan if preferred). While assembling the food on 2 plates, wilt the spinach in the pan.

- **CALORIES** 330
- PROTEIN 19G
- FAT 24G
- FIBRE 2G
- CARBS 9G

Quick Lunches, Smart Snacks

The people who do really well on the Blood Sugar Diet tend to be those who have identified the moments at which they are at greatest risk of breaking their good intentions. For some, this is on days when they are trying to skip lunch; for others, it is when they get back from work and need something to take the edge off their hunger. This is Michael's Achilles heel – how to avoid going for the toast…

Remember, successful dieting is less about will power than good planning. We recommend having a small portion of something tasty – a dip, nibble, healthy seed bar – ready to hand when you need it, to keep temptation at bay.

That said, we would urge you as far as possible to try and avoid snacking between meals. It's when you haven't eaten for a while that you burn fat and flush out the sugar stored in your liver and pancreas. As soon as you snack, you stop that restorative process in its tracks.

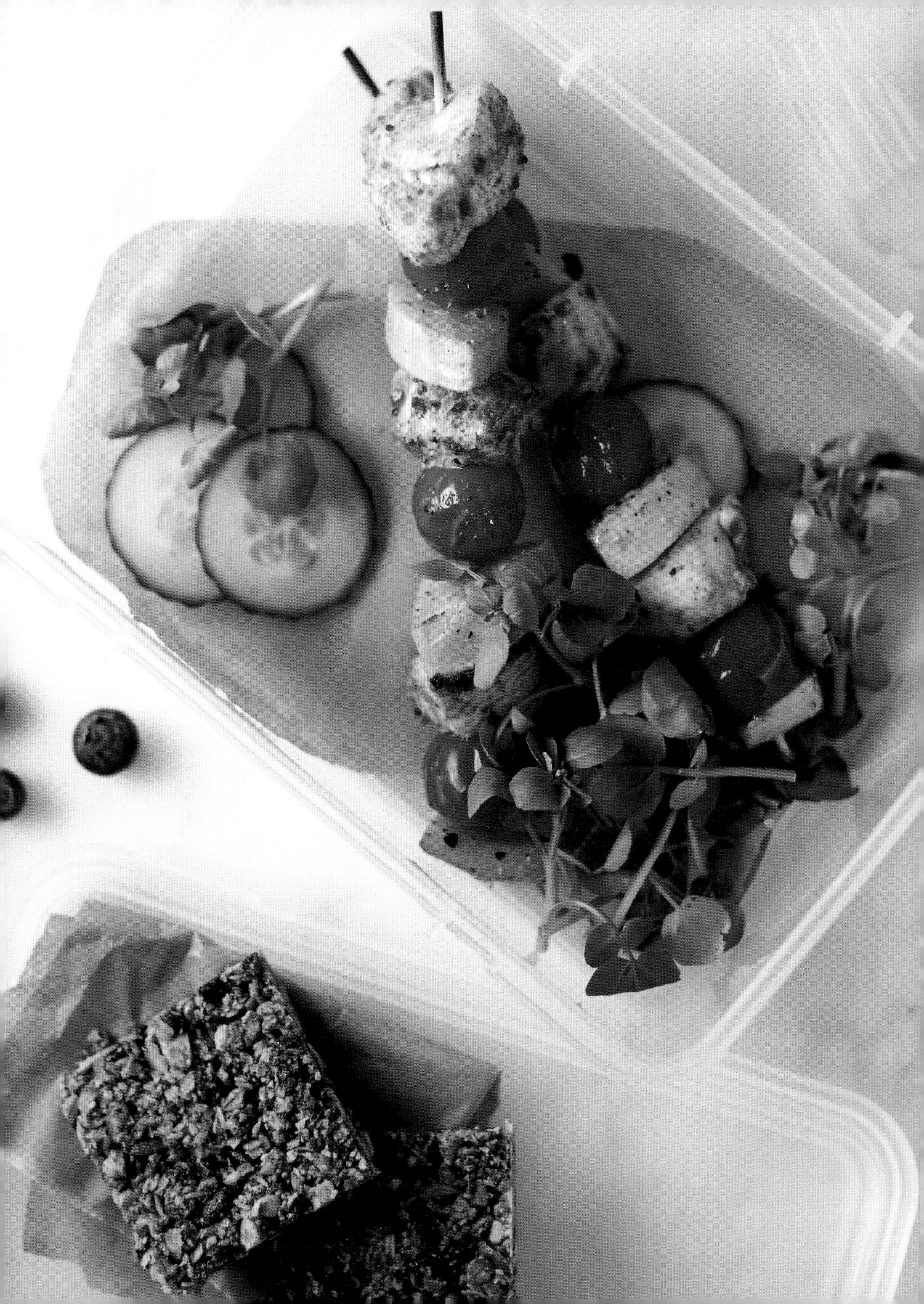

Quick lunches

It can be a struggle to find healthy food to eat on the go. Here are some yummy alternatives to the standard sandwich or pie – simple, portable kebabs, soups and salads that not only taste great, but will fill you up, too.

Taco lettuce wrap 4 ways

This is a skinny version of a wrap, using crisp cos or little gem lettuce instead of a starchy taco or tortilla. For a packed lunch, simply wrap the filled lettuce leaves in clingfilm or foil, as you would a sandwich.

1. Salmon and avocado

Serves 1

1 avocado
4 outer leaves from a gem lettuce (or cos)
100g smoked salmon
Squeeze of lemon juice
1 tsp sesame seeds

Mash the avocado and dollop it into the base of the lettuce leaves. Add a strip of smoked salmon, a squeeze of lemon, a grinding of black pepper and scatter with the sesame seeds.

- CALORIES 470
- PROTEIN 26G
- FAT 50G
- FIBRE 7G
- CARBS 5G

2. Tuna and tomato salsa

Serves 1

80g tin tuna, drained
2 tomatoes, finely diced
¼ red onion, finely diced
Dash of Tabasco
Squeeze of lime juice
4 outer leaves from a gem lettuce (or cos)
Handful of coriander, chopped

Mix the tuna in a bowl with the tomatoes, red onion, Tabasco, lime juice and some black pepper. Divide the mixture between the 4 lettuce leaves. Garnish with coriander.

- **CALORIES** 140
- PROTEIN 26G
- FAT 2G
- FIBRE 3G
- CARBS 7G

---

3. Feta and avocado bash

Serves 1

1 avocado
30g feta
Squeeze of lime juice
4 outer leaves from a gem lettuce (or cos)
Handful of parsley, chopped

Place the avocado and feta in a bowl and use a fork or potato masher to blend them together, then stir in the lime juice. Divide the mixture between the 4 lettuce leaves, season with freshly ground black pepper and sprinkle on the parsley.

- **CALORIES** 370
- PROTEIN 8G
- FAT 35G
- FIBRE 6G
- CARBS 5G

---

4. Roast peppers with hummus and nuts

Serves 1

3 strips of roasted red pepper from a jar, chopped
2 heaped tbsp hummus
4 outer leaves from a gem lettuce (or cos)
2 tsp pine nuts

Mix the strips of pepper with the hummus in a bowl. Season with a pinch of salt and black pepper. Divide the mixture between the 4 lettuce leaves and sprinkle on the pine nuts.

- **CALORIES** 190
- PROTEIN 7G
- FAT 15G
- FIBRE 2G
- CARBS 10G

Instant salads

Many people now take a salad in a box to work for their lunch. The salads below all work well assembled in advance. Find a small pot for the dressing (with a good seal so it doesn't leak!) and store the salad in a separate container to keep it crisp and fresh.

Lentil and feta salad

Lentils are a key part of the Mediterranean diet, containing plenty of fibre and protein to help keep you feeling fuller for longer. They are also a good source of iron.

Serves 2

½ 400g tin black or green lentils, drained
1 spring onion, finely sliced
60g feta or Cheddar, crumbled
Handful of parsley, chopped
Handful of salad leaves, such as rocket or crispy cos.
½ tsp dried herbs, such as thyme or oregano
Pinch of chilli flakes

For the dressing:
1 tbsp balsamic vinegar
2 tbsp extra-virgin olive oil

Mix all the ingredients together in a bowl, and season to taste. Whisk together the oil and vinegar to make the dressing and drizzle it over the salad.

Tip: if preparing for one, the second portion will keep in the fridge for a couple of days.

- CALORIES 290
- PROTEIN 7G
- FAT 14G
- FIBRE 3G
- CARBS 11G

Greek salad

The ultimate in Mediterranean-style food, a Greek salad makes a perfect light lunch, and also works well as a side dish for a main meal. Buy the very best vegetables you can – ripe tomatoes, good olives, fresh mint – and ideally serve at room temperature to get the most out of their flavours.

Serves 2

4 medium, vine-ripened tomatoes, chopped
½ cucumber, deseeded and roughly chopped
½ red onion, thinly sliced
8 black olives, stoned and halved
60g feta, diced
Handful of mint leaves, chopped

For the dressing:
2 tbsp extra-virgin olive oil
Juice of half a lemon
½ tsp dried oregano

Toss all the ingredients in a bowl. Whisk together the dressing ingredients and drizzle it over the salad. Summer holiday on a plate.

- **CALORIES** 250
- PROTEIN 5G
- FAT 15G
- FIBRE 3G
- CARBS 10G

Tuna, artichoke and butterbean salad

Artichokes are not only tasty, they are packed with wonderful nutrients and phytochemicals. They are so good for your gut bacteria that they are known as prebiotics.

Serves 2

200g tin tuna, drained
2 spring onions, chopped
8 cherry tomatoes, halved
400g tin butterbeans, drained and rinsed
2 artichoke hearts from a jar, quartered

For the dressing:
2 tbsp olive oil
Juice of half a lemon
1 tsp Dijon mustard
Handful of parsley leaves, chopped

Place the tuna in a bowl and break it up into chunks. Add the spring onions, tomatoes, beans and artichokes and toss everything together. Whisk together the dressing ingredients and drizzle it over the salad.

Tip: olive oil, like avocados and most nuts, contains large amounts of oleic acid and is a health-promoting staple of the Mediterranean diet. Enjoy it. Drizzle it on your salads, over hummus, on vegetables, beans and pulses...

- **CALORIES** 410
- PROTEIN 40G
- FAT 16G
- FIBRE 10G
- CARBS 30G

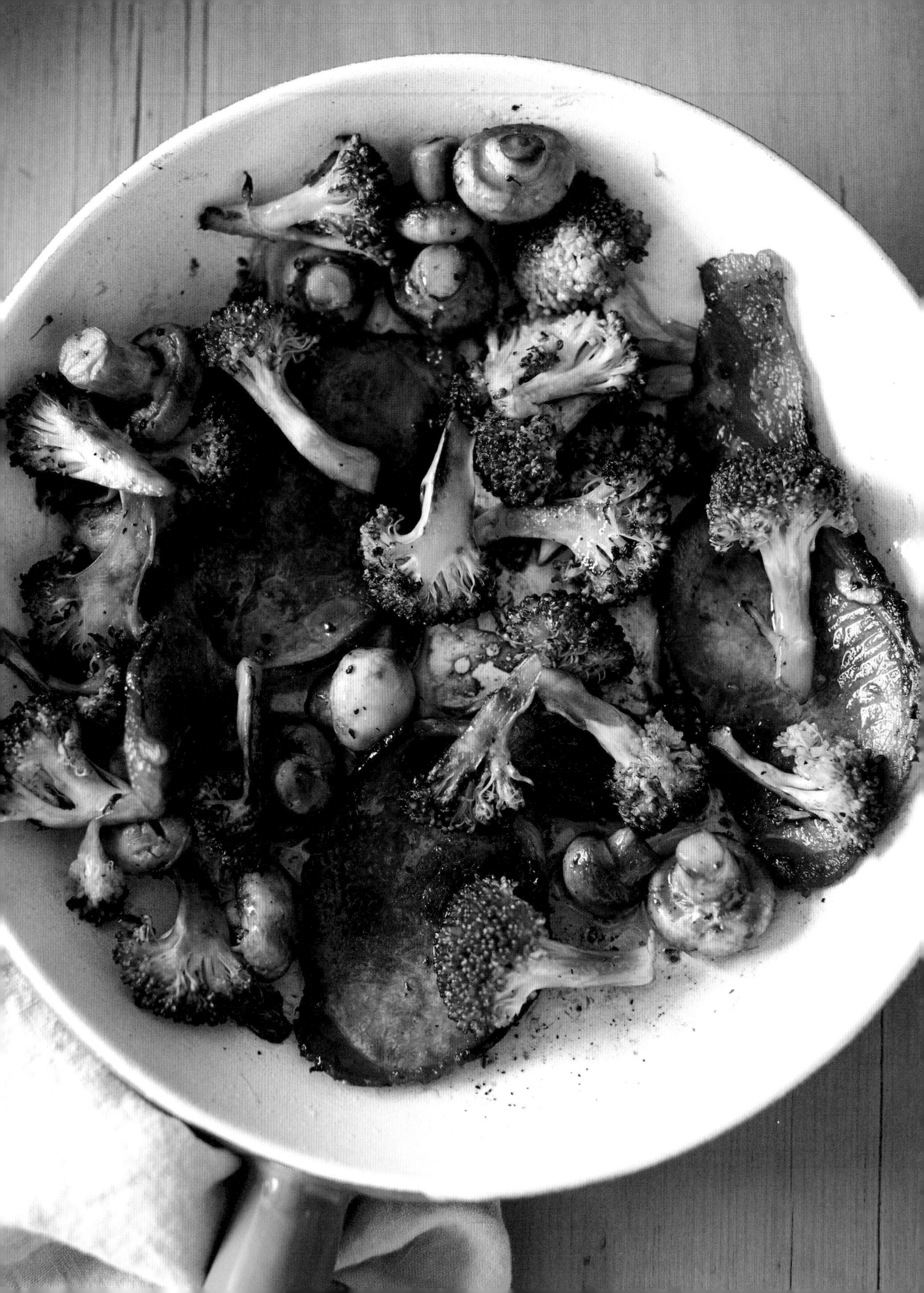

Dr David Unwin's quick bacon and broccoli fry-up

A delicious, easy lunch, kindly sent to us by the inspirational GP Dr David Unwin, who has been championing the low-carb, higher-fat approach to eating for some years. He has helped many of his patients lose weight, improve their blood sugars and reverse their diabetes; and was doing this at a time when people didn't believe it was possible.

Serves 1

3 rashers of bacon, diced
1 tbsp olive oil
100g button mushrooms
200g broccoli, roughly chopped, or leeks, sliced
20g cheese, grated

Fry the bacon in the olive oil, add the mushrooms and then the broccoli and cook until everything has softened and melded together. Add some black pepper and sprinkle on the grated cheese, and tuck in. (Even better, if you have time: place the mixture in an oven dish under the grill until it's golden brown on top.)

Tip: you can replace the bacon with either 60g halloumi, fried first like the bacon, or 80g peppered mackerel, which should be added at the end to the softened veg mixture.

- **CALORIES** 430
- PROTEIN 29G
- FAT 33G
- FIBRE 6G
- CARBS 4G

Speedy spicy beans

This vegetarian dish – inspired by a recipe from Hashimoto on the Blood Sugar Diet website – is fabulously easy to make and is ready in 5 minutes.

Serves 1

½ red onion or shallot, chopped
½ tbsp olive oil
½ red pepper, deseeded and chopped
½ medium courgette, diced into 2cm pieces
1 garlic clove, chopped or crushed
1 chilli, deseeded and sliced, or 1 tsp chilli flakes
½ 415g tin reduced-sugar baked beans
Splash of Worcestershire sauce (optional)

In a medium-sized pan, sweat the onion in the oil for a few minutes. Add the pepper, courgette, garlic and chilli, and cook for another few minutes until the veg have slightly softened. Stir in the baked beans and Worcestershire sauce and make sure everything is thoroughly heated through before serving.

Tip: on a non-fast day you could add a slice of the seeded spelt and rye bread (see page 181).

- **CALORIES** 250
- PROTEIN 12G
- FAT 7G
- FIBRE 9G
- CARBS 37G

Runner beans with halloumi

A wonderfully crisp, green summer dish, which is also infinitely adaptable.

Serves 2

80g halloumi cheese (or 4 rashers of bacon, chopped)
1 tbsp olive oil
250g runner beans (or other seasonal veg, such as mange tout or sugar snap peas), trimmed and diced
1 tbsp pecorino (or Parmesan), grated
Handful of pine nuts (or other seeds), toasted

Fry the halloumi (or the bacon, if using) in the oil. Steam, boil or microwave the beans so they are still a bit crunchy. In a bowl, mix the hot beans with the halloumi and the pecorino. Season with black pepper and sprinkle the toasted pine nuts over before serving.

- **CALORIES** 320
- PROTEIN 17G
- FAT 26G
- FIBRE 3G
- CARBS 6G

Omelette 2 ways

1. Japanese omelette

Serves 1

2 eggs
½ tbsp soy sauce
50g cabbage or greens, finely chopped (or use leftover greens)
1 tbsp coconut oil or light olive oil
½ tsp root ginger, finely chopped
¼ tsp chilli flakes
2-3 spring onions, finely diced
Small handful of coriander leaves, chopped
Sushi pickled ginger from a jar (optional)

Whisk the eggs with the soy sauce. Steam, microwave or boil the greens for a couple of minutes, so they are tender but still crisp. In a small frying pan, heat the oil and add the diced ginger, chilli and spring onions. Fry them gently for about a minute, then pour in the eggs. Immediately add the greens and coriander and cook the omelette gently until the underside is golden brown. Fold it in half and serve it while it is still a bit runny, with sushi pickled ginger, if using, and a grating of black pepper.

- **CALORIES** 270
- PROTEIN 14G
- FAT 21G
- FIBRE 2G
- CARBS 5G

---

2. Cheese and asparagus omelette

This is Michael's absolute favourite, sprinkled liberally with chilli flakes for an extra kick.

Serves 1

3-4 asparagus spears, halved lengthwise and cut into 3cm pieces
Knob of butter
2 eggs, beaten
20g strong Cheddar, grated
5g Parmesan, grated
Pinch of chilli flakes (optional)

Steam the asparagus for 1½ minutes (or less if using a microwave). In a small non-stick frying pan, melt the butter, then pour in the eggs and cook them over a gentle heat. Scatter the Cheddar and Parmesan over the surface and add the asparagus. When the surface is still a little bit soft, fold the omelette in half. Season and sprinkle with chilli flakes, if using.

- **CALORIES** 290
- PROTEIN 23G
- FAT 22G
- FIBRE 1G
- CARBS 1G

Kebabs to go

These make delicious, healthy snacks on a stick. With a bit of planning you can have them ready to take to work. Buy a pack of short wooden sticks that fit into your lunch box. For kebabs made of meat or fish, it would be wise to include a small ice pack in the box if you are going to be out for more than an hour or two in the heat.

In the ideal world you would cook them over a barbecue, but they still taste superb done under a hot grill or on a griddle.

1. Lemon prawn kebabs

Serves 1

2 tbsp olive oil
Juice of 1 lemon
12 king prawns, fresh or frozen (defrosted)
12 cherry tomatoes
3 asparagus spears, cut into 4 pieces
3 wooden skewers, soaked in water

Place the oil in a bowl, mix in the lemon juice and season well with salt and plenty of black pepper. Then add the prawns, tomatoes and asparagus and toss everything so it gets a good coating. Thread the prawns and veg onto the skewers and place them under a hot grill for 10 minutes, turning frequently. Serve with a dollop of Greek yoghurt (add 30 calories).

- **CALORIES** 360
- PROTEIN 21G
- FAT 28G
- FIBRE 3G
- CARBS 7G

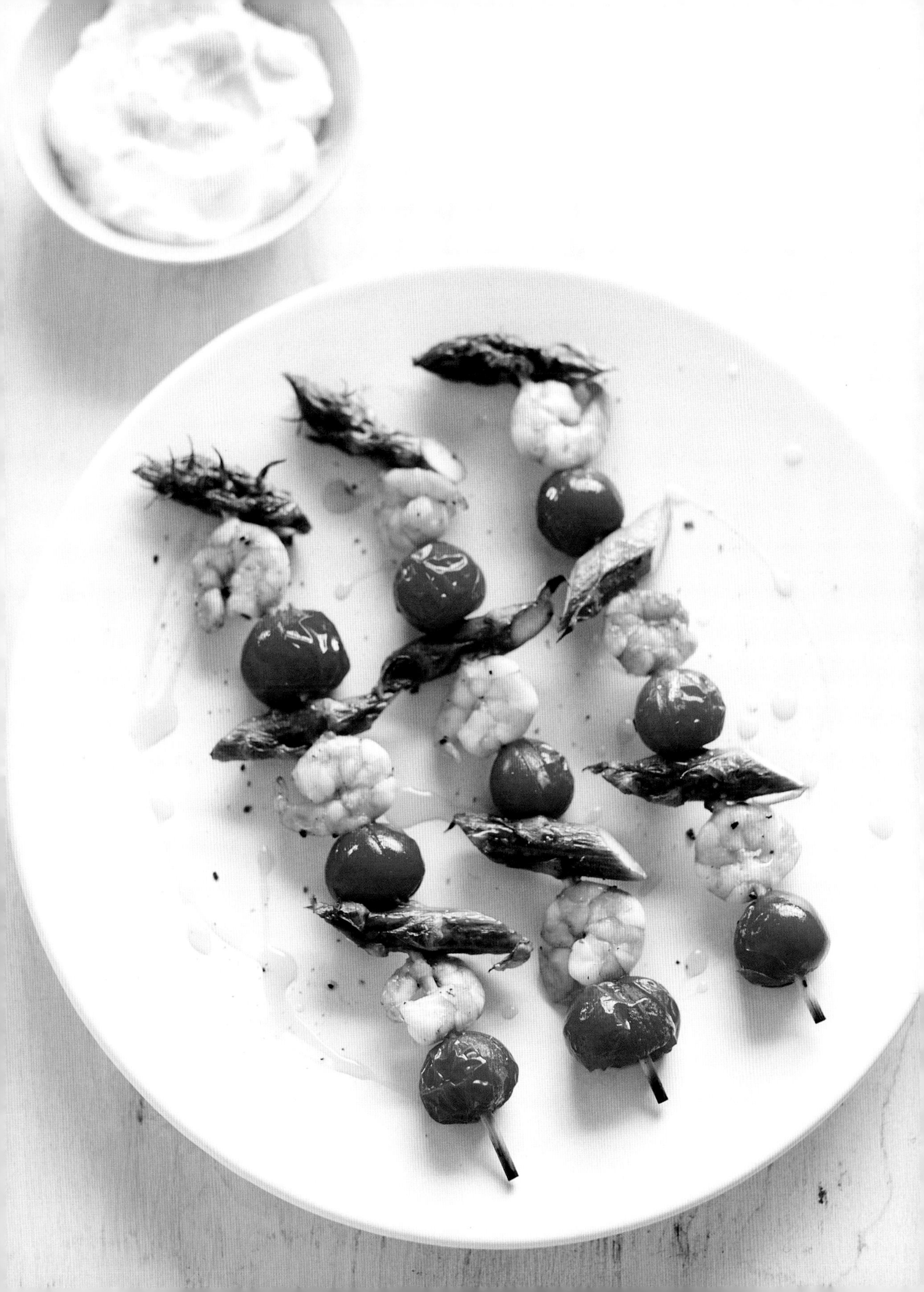

2. Halloumi kebabs

Serves 1

90g halloumi
6 artichoke hearts from a jar
1 red pepper
2 tbsp olive oil
1 tsp ras el hanout (or paprika)
3 wooden skewers, soaked in water

Dice the halloumi into 9 cubes, halve the artichoke hearts and chop the pepper into 12 pieces. Put them in a bowl with the oil and spice and some seasoning, and toss everything well so it gets a good coating. Thread the kebab pieces onto the skewers, then place them under a hot grill for 5-6 minutes, turning frequently. Serve with low-sugar sweet chilli sauce (see page 175) or raitha (see page 72).

- **CALORIES** 430
- PROTEIN 19G
- FAT 34G
- FIBRE 3G
- CARBS 15G

---

3. Ploughman's on a stick

I like to think of this as a tasty low-carb version of what you might get in a pub. Choose your favourite cheese – just make sure it is not too runny or crumbly, so that it stays on the stick. For variation, you could add a few rolls of salami or ham.

Serves 1

3 slices of ham, cut into strips and rolled
9 silverskin cocktail onions (or small gherkins)
1 apple, cored and chopped into chunks
60g Cheddar, diced
3 wooden skewers
1 tbsp pickle

Thread the ham, onions, apple and cheese onto the skewers. Serve with the pickle.

- **CALORIES** 400
- PROTEIN 24G
- FAT 25G
- FIBRE 2G
- CARBS 18G

4. Spiced lamb kebabs

Serves 1

100g lamb steak
1 green pepper, deseeded
2 tbsp olive oil
2 tsp harissa paste (or curry paste)
12 button mushrooms
3 wooden skewers, soaked in water

Dice the lamb and pepper into 12 pieces. Pour the oil into a bowl and stir in the harissa paste. Add the lamb and mix well. If you have time, leave it to marinate for a few hours. Then add the pepper and mushrooms and stir well so everything gets a good coating. Thread the kebab pieces onto the skewers, alternating the lamb, pepper and mushrooms. Place them under a hot grill for 10 minutes, turning frequently. Serve with raitha or tzatziki (see page 72).

- **CALORIES** 460
- PROTEIN 32G
- FAT 45G
- FIBRE 5G
- CARBS 8G

---

5. Paprika chicken kebab

Serves 1

1 skinless chicken breast
1 tbsp olive oil, plus a little extra for drizzling
1 garlic clove, crushed
1 tsp paprika
Juice of half a lemon
Pinch of chilli flakes (optional)
1 courgette
1 red onion, quartered
3 wooden skewers, soaked in water

Slice the chicken breast into 3 long strips and then dice each strip, aiming to get about 12 cubes. Mix the oil in a bowl with the garlic, paprika, lemon juice, chilli flakes, if using, and some seasoning, and then add the chicken, tossing everything together so it gets a good coating. Chop the courgette into 12 chunks and then cut the onion quarters into three so you have 12 chunks of that too. Toss the courgette and onion in a bowl with a drizzle of oil and some salt and pepper.

Thread the kebab pieces onto the skewers, alternating the chicken, courgette and onion. Place them under a hot grill for 12-15 minutes, turning every 3-4 minutes. Serve with tzatziki (see page 72).

- **CALORIES** 190
- PROTEIN 12G
- FAT 14G
- FIBRE 1G
- CARBS 6G

6. Piri piri chicken sticks

Serves 1

1 skinless chicken breast
2 tbsp olive oil
1 tsp piri piri seasoning
12 cherry tomatoes
¼ butternut squash, peeled and cubed (or 12 pieces of shop-bought, ready-chopped)
3 wooden skewers, soaked in water

Slice the chicken breast into three long strips and then dice each strip, aiming to get 12 cubes. Mix 1 tbsp oil and the piri piri seasoning in a bowl, then add the chicken, tossing it well so it gets a good coating. Leave it to marinate for a few hours, if time permits.

Toss the tomatoes and butternut squash in a separate bowl with the remaining oil and some salt and pepper. Thread the kebab pieces onto the skewers, alternating the chicken, tomato and squash. Place them under a hot grill for 12-15 minutes, turning every 3-4 minutes. Serve with raitha (see page 72).

Tip: to make your own piri piri flavouring, mix together 1 tsp paprika, 1 tsp oregano, 1-2 fresh chillies, deseeded and diced (or 1-2 tsp chilli flakes), and 1 tsp garlic, either paste or a finely chopped clove.

- **CALORIES** 360
- PROTEIN 13G
- FAT 28G
- FIBRE 4G
- CARBS 18G

---

7. Chinese tofu kebabs

Serves 1

120g tofu
2 spring onions
1 red pepper, deseeded
1 tbsp olive oil
Juice of half a lime
1 tsp Chinese 5-spice
1 tsp soy sauce
1 tsp fish sauce
3 wooden skewers, soaked in water

Dice the tofu into 12 cubes, cut each spring onion into 6 pieces and the pepper into 12. Mix the oil in a bowl with the lime juice, spice, soy and fish sauce and then add the tofu, spring onions and pepper, tossing everything well so it gets a good coating. Thread the skewers, alternating ingredients, and place them under a hot grill for 10 minutes, turning frequently. Serve with low-sugar sweet chilli sauce (see page 175).

- **CALORIES** 230
- PROTEIN 12G
- FAT 16G
- FIBRE 3G
- CARBS 12G

8. Satay chicken kebabs

An exotic South East Asian mix. Irresistible.

Serves 2

2 skinless chicken breasts
1 garlic clove, crushed
½ red chilli, deseeded and chopped
2 tbsp soy sauce
1 tbsp coconut oil
6 wooden skewers, soaked in water

For the satay sauce:
2 tbsp coconut oil
2 spring onions, diced
1 garlic clove, crushed
½ red chilli, deseeded and chopped
3 tbsp peanut butter
½ tbsp fish sauce
100ml coconut milk

To make the kebabs, slice each chicken breast into 3 long strips and then dice each strip, aiming to get 12-15 cubes from each. Make a marinade in a bowl by mixing together the garlic and chilli, soy sauce and coconut oil. Toss the chicken pieces in the marinade, making sure they are well coated. Cover them with clingfilm and leave them in the fridge overnight.

When you are ready to eat, thread 4 or 5 cubes onto each wooden skewer, season them with salt and pepper and place them under a hot grill for 12-15 minutes, turning every 3-4 minutes.

Meanwhile, to make the sauce, put a pan on a medium heat, add the coconut oil and fry the spring onions, garlic and chilli for 3-4 minutes or until they are soft. Add the peanut butter and fish sauce and keep stirring for another 2 minutes. Transfer the mixture to a food processor, add the coconut milk and blend to a smooth paste.

Taste the sauce and add a splash of soy sauce if you wish. Serve the kebabs on a bed of rocket with the dipping sauce on the side.

- **CALORIES** 460
- PROTEIN 33G
- FAT 44G
- FIBRE 2G
- CARBS 10G

Soups

Soup not only makes a delicious meal, it can be very filling. Studies have shown that eating food blended into a soup keeps you satisfied for longer, compared with eating the same food separately along with the extra fluid. We suggest making enough for 4 portions so that you can put anything left over in the freezer for instant sustenance another day.

Celeriac and apple soup

Serves 4

1 tbsp olive oil
1 onion, chopped
1 leek, sliced
2cm root ginger, chopped
1 celeriac, peeled and chopped
4 eating apples, cored and quartered
Large pinch of thyme leaves
2 litres vegetable or chicken stock
200ml crème fraîche
1 tbsp nuts, chopped

Heat the oil in a large saucepan. Add the onion, leek and ginger and cook them over a medium heat for 10 minutes until they are soft. Stir in the celeriac, apples and thyme and cook for a few more minutes. Pour in the stock and some seasoning and simmer for 30 minutes. When the celeriac is tender, remove the soup from the heat and use a hand blender (or a food processor) to blitz it until it is smooth. Stir in half the crème fraîche, reserving the remainder to dollop into each bowl. Serve with a scattering of chopped nuts.

- CALORIES 320
- PROTEIN 5G
- FAT 24G
- FIBRE 8G
- CARBS 20G

Chicken lime laksa

Serves 4

Bunch of fresh coriander
Drizzle of olive oil
4 spring onions, sliced
1 red pepper, deseeded and sliced
1 tsp chilli paste
1 tsp ginger paste
1 tsp Chinese 5-spice
1 pack (approx 300g) of ready-chopped butternut squash
1.2 litres chicken or vegetable stock
Juice of 2 limes
1 tbsp soy sauce
1 tbsp Thai fish sauce
300g cooked chicken, diced
400g green beans
400ml tin of coconut milk
2 large handfuls of baby spinach leaves (or fresh greens, chopped)

Chop off the coriander stalks, retaining the leaves. Heat the oil in a large saucepan and fry the stalks, spring onions, pepper, chilli, ginger paste and Chinese 5 spice on a medium heat for 2-3 minutes. Add the butternut squash and cook for a further 2 minutes, then pour in the stock, lime juice, soy and fish sauces and bring the mixture to the boil. Turn down the heat and simmer for 10 minutes. Add the chicken, beans, coconut milk and spinach and cook until the beans have softened and the chicken has warmed through. Serve topped with the coriander leaves.

- **CALORIES** 330
- PROTEIN 21G
- FAT 23G
- FIBRE 2G
- CARBS 9G

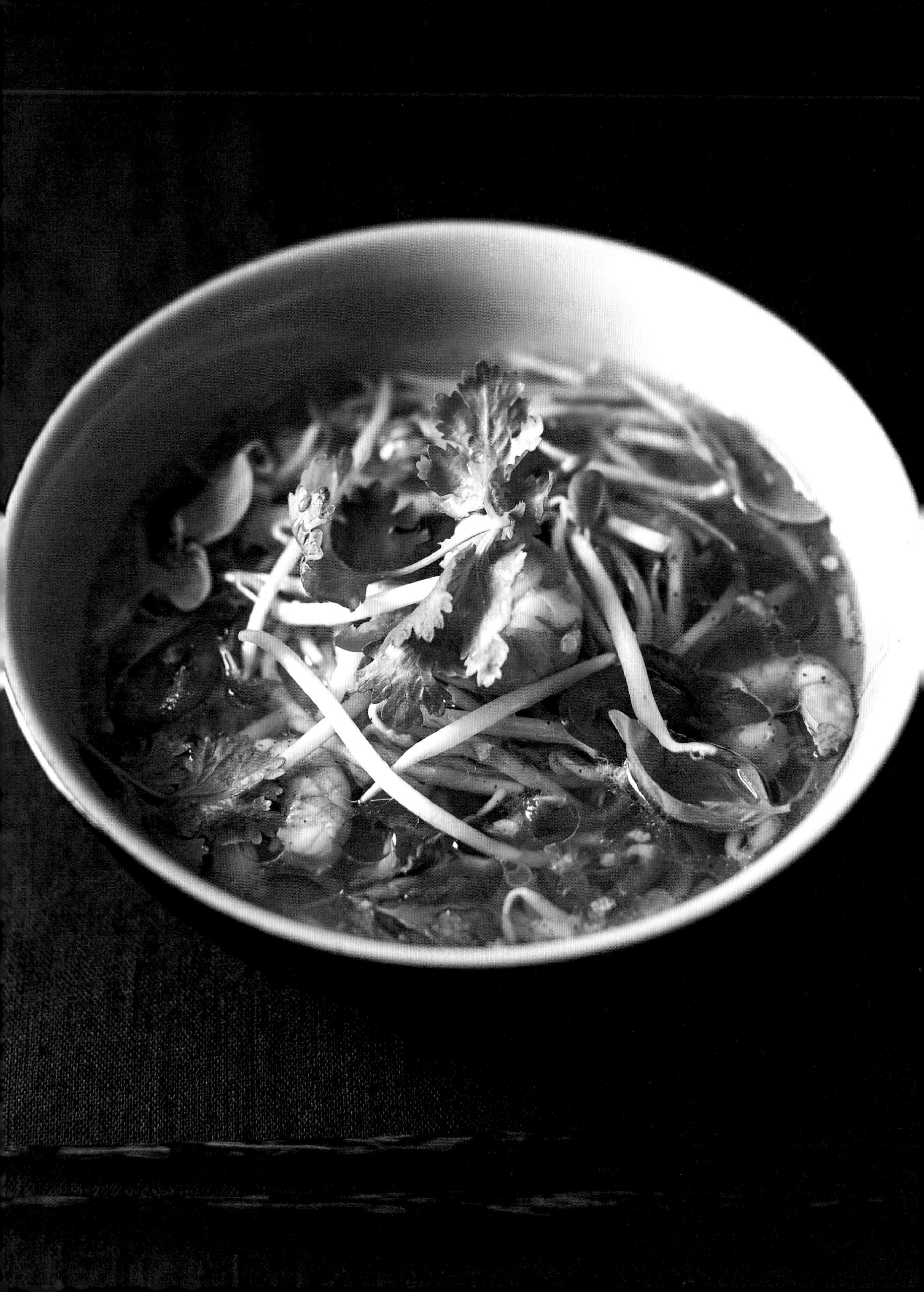

Vietnamese pho

This soup makes a wonderful light lunch. The low-carb konjac noodles add few calories to the dish. They are made from yams and have been eaten in Japan for centuries.

Serves 2

2 tsp coconut oil
2cm root ginger, grated
2 spring onions, chopped
1 litre vegetable stock
Juice of 1 lime
1 tbsp Thai fish sauce
1 tbsp mirin or cider vinegar
8 large prawns (fresh or frozen)
1 bag of beansprouts
50g spring greens, shredded
100g konjac noodles, rinsed and drained (optional, see tip)
Handful of fresh basil or coriander
½ red chilli, deseeded and finely sliced (or pinch of chilli flakes)

Heat the coconut oil in a large saucepan, and fry the ginger and spring onions for 2-3 minutes. Pour in the stock, add the lime juice, fish sauce and mirin and season with salt and pepper. Bring the mixture to the boil and simmer for 10 minutes. Add the prawns and cook them for 5 minutes more, or until they turn pink. Then add the beansprouts, greens and konjac noodles, if using. Serve the pho with the herbs and chilli scattered over.

Tip: if konjac noodles are not available, you might substitute 100g courgetti spaghetti (see page 107), or skip them altogether as the beansprouts provide plenty of texture. You can also replace the prawns with tofu, chicken or beef.

- **CALORIES** 120
- PROTEIN 13G
- FAT 7G
- FIBRE 2G
- CARBS 7G

Tomato, ham and lentil soup

A favourite, comforting soup, often to be found bubbling away when we visit Michael's mum.

Serves 4

2 tbsp olive oil
1 onion, chopped
1 red pepper, deseeded and chopped
1 garlic clove, crushed
1 tsp chilli flakes
175g red lentils
2 x 400g tins chopped tomatoes
1.5 litres vegetable or chicken stock
200g leftover ham (or bacon or pancetta), chopped
2 tbsp parsley or coriander, chopped
200g pot sour cream and chive dip (full-fat)

Heat the oil in a large saucepan and gently fry the onion and pepper for 6-8 minutes. Add the garlic and chilli and stir for a minute, then tip in the lentils, tomatoes and stock. Bring the pan to the boil, cover it and leave it to simmer for 30 minutes or until the lentils are really tender and beginning to break up. Stir in the ham and herbs and season to taste, then remove the soup from the heat and mash it roughly with a potato masher, leaving some texture. Serve each portion with 1 tbsp of the sour cream and chive dip.

- CALORIES 440
- PROTEIN 25G
- FAT 23G
- FIBRE 5G
- CARBS 40G

Miso soup

Miso soup is made from fermented soya beans with a base of dashi, a Japanese broth of seaweed and dried fish. Michael lived on this (without any of the extras), when he did a 4-day fast prior to starting the 5:2 Fast Diet. He found it a lifeline and looked forward to it – warm and tasty and very low in calories.

Serves 1

300ml dashi stock
2 tbsp miso paste
1 spring onion, finely chopped
1cm root ginger, grated
1 tbsp mirin

Mix 1 tbsp dashi stock with the miso paste to dissolve it. Heat the remaining stock in a saucepan and stir in the loosened paste, bring it to the boil and allow it to simmer for 10 minutes. Add the spring onion and ginger and simmer for a further 2-3 minutes.

- **CALORIES** 90
- PROTEIN 6G
- FAT 3G
- FIBRE 0G
- CARBS 11G

For a more substantial version, choose a handful of any of the following, each about 10 calories, unless stated: Chinese cabbage, pak choi, broccoli, any leafy green veg, tinned water chestnuts, bamboo shoots, beansprouts, grated or spiralised carrot, finely chopped leeks or shiitake mushrooms (add 20 calories for these). Simmer the veg in the stock for about 5 minutes, depending on how crunchy you like them.

For a shot of protein, you could also add: a raw egg, cracked in to poach for 3-5 minutes; or 50g any cooked fish or meat, such as pork, turkey, chicken, poached salmon or crab (add 90 calories); or 100g tempeh, tofu or prawns (add approx 100 calories).

For a more exotic option, top with kaiso (dried seaweed, which rehydrates in hot liquid) or nori (shredded seaweed). You could also add a little sushi pickled ginger from a jar.

Roasted red pepper and squash soup

Serves 4

4 red or orange peppers, halved and deseeded
½ large butternut squash, peeled and diced (or 400-500g bag of ready prepared)
1 onion, diced
2 tbsp olive oil
1 litre vegetable stock
½ tsp chilli flakes (or ½ red chilli, deseeded and diced)
Handful of parsley or coriander, chopped

Preheat the oven to 180°C. Spread the peppers, squash and onion on a large oven tray. Season them and drizzle over 1 tbsp olive oil. Bake the veg in the oven until the edges begin to blacken (about 20 minutes). When the peppers have cooled sufficiently, remove most of the skin and roughly chop them.

Heat the rest of the olive oil in a large saucepan and put in the baked vegetables. Add the stock and chilli flakes and bring it to the boil, then leave it to simmer for about 20 minutes or until everything is soft. Remove the pan from the heat and blend the soup with a hand blender or food processor. Bring it back to the boil before serving it garnished with the parsley or coriander. (For a richer dish, you can add a handful of fried chorizo; alternatively, add 1 tbsp each of fried diced halloumi or toasted nuts – see page 177.)

- **CALORIES** 150
- PROTEIN 3G
- FAT 6G
- FIBRE 4G
- CARBS 22G

Gazpacho

A simple summer classic.

Serves 4

2 x 400g tins chopped tomatoes
½ cucumber, deseeded and cut into chunks
1 garlic clove, finely chopped
1 red pepper, deseeded and chopped
2 tbsp olive oil
3 tbsp cider vinegar (or red wine vinegar)
Handful of basil leaves
12 ice cubes

Tip the tomatoes into a food processor, followed by the cucumber, garlic, red pepper, olive oil, vinegar and most of the the basil. Season with salt and freshly ground black pepper. Add a few ice cubes, a drizzle of olive oil and a sprinkling of shredded basil leaves to each bowl before serving.

- **CALORIES** 100
- PROTEIN 3G
- FAT 5G
- FIBRE 8G
- CARBS 10G

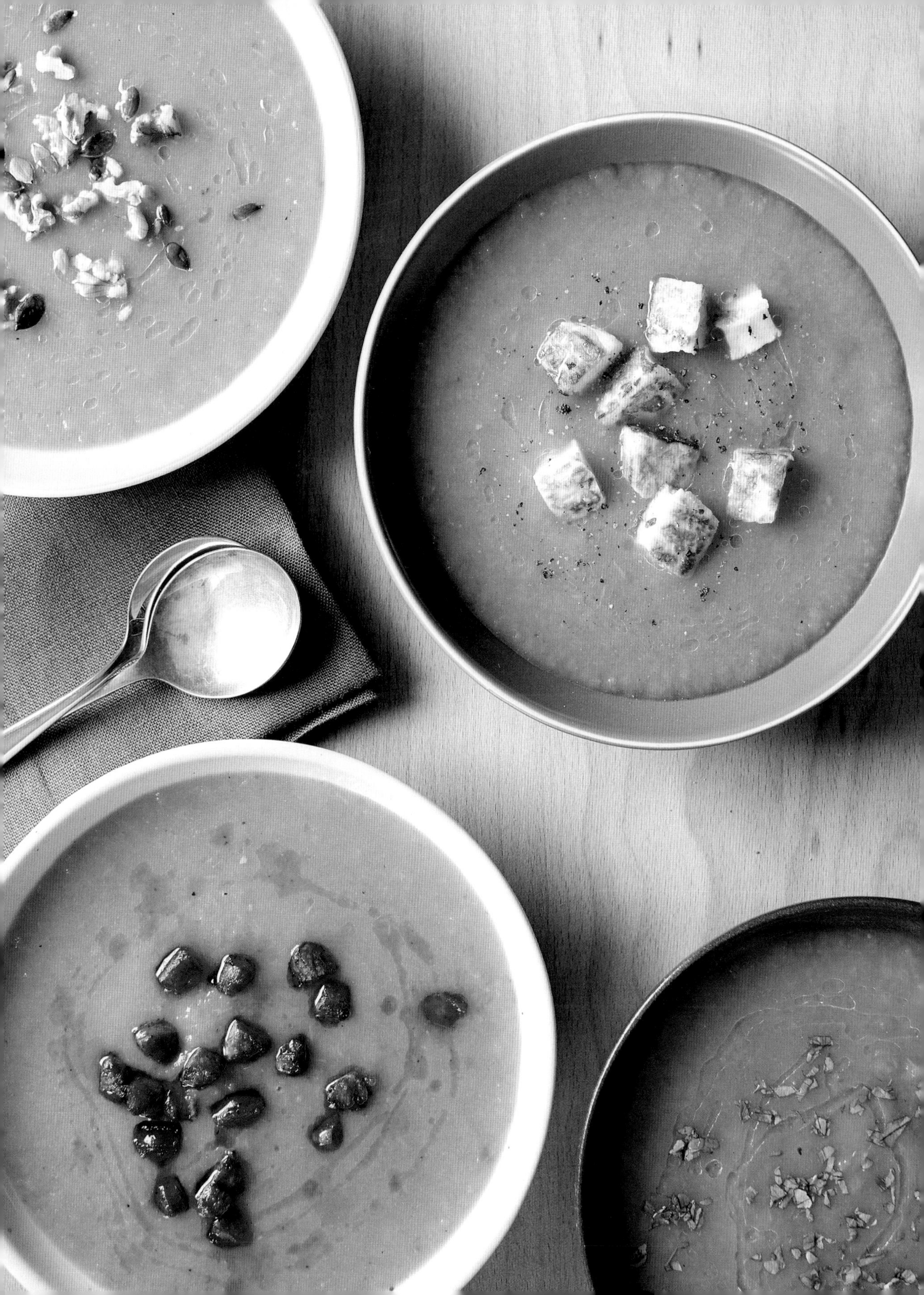

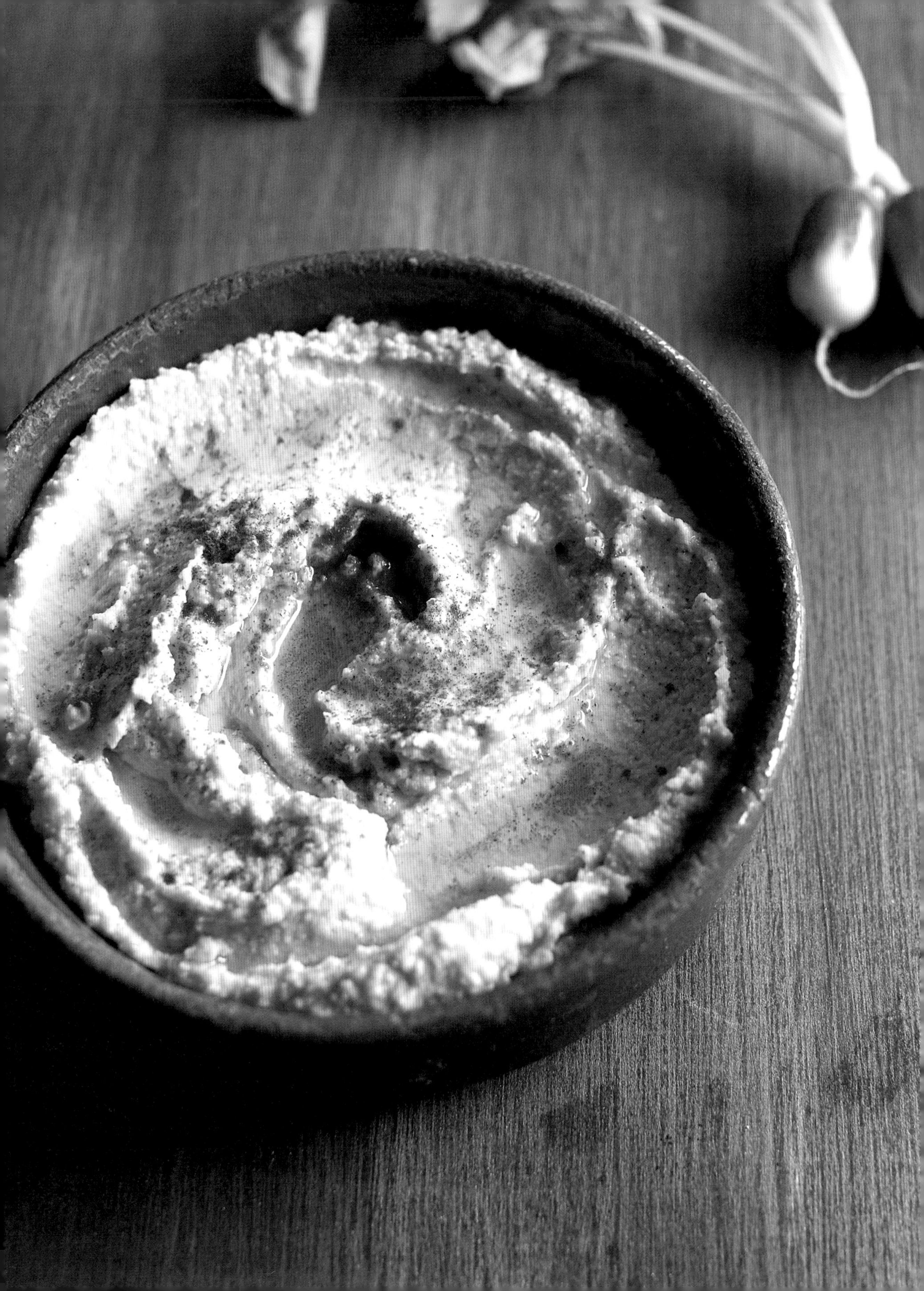

Smart snacks

A range of tasty, filling dips and nibbles which will have minimal impact on blood sugars.

Skinny dips

The following dips can be served as accompaniments to almost any meal. For a light lunch, have a portion with batons or chunks of any crunchy, salad-type vegetable as a delicious alternative to crisps, bread and pitta.

Perfect hummus

Makes 4 portions

400g tin chickpeas, drained and rinsed
3 tbsp lemon juice (or more, to taste)
6 tbsp extra-virgin olive oil
4 tsp tahini
2 garlic cloves, crushed
1 tsp ground cumin
Pinch of salt
3 tbsp water, as required
1 tsp paprika

Blend the chickpeas, lemon juice, olive oil, tahini, garlic, cumin, salt and water in a food processor until you have a creamy purée. Serve it with a drizzle of olive oil and a sprinkling of paprika.

- CALORIES 210
- PROTEIN 9G
- FAT 13G
- FIBRE 5G
- CARBS 17G

Tzatziki

Makes 4 portions

2 small cucumbers
300ml full-fat Greek yogurt
Juice of 1 lemon
2-3 garlic cloves, finely grated
1 tbsp olive oil
1 tsp paprika

Peel and deseed the cucumbers, then grate or finely dice them. Combine them in a bowl with the yoghurt and all the other ingredients and a pinch of salt and black pepper.

- **CALORIES** 140
- PROTEIN 4G
- FAT 1G
- FIBRE 0G
- CARBS 4G

Raitha

This makes a great dip, as well as a tasty accompaniment to a curry.

Makes 4 portions

½ cucumber
250ml full-fat Greek yoghurt
¼ tsp cumin seeds
2-3 mint leaves, finely chopped

Peel and deseed the cucumber, then grate or finely dice it. Combine it in a bowl with the yoghurt and all the other ingredients and a large pinch of salt.

- **CALORIES** 80
- PROTEIN 4G
- FAT 6G
- FIBRE 0G
- CARBS 2G

Smoked fish paté

Makes 2 portions

1 fillet smoked mackerel (or trout)
3 tbsp full-fat soft cheese
Squeeze of lemon juice
1-2 tsp hot horseradish sauce
½ cucumber, thickly sliced

Remove the skin from the mackerel fillet and mash the fish in a bowl with the cheese and lemon juice. Season the mixture with black pepper, and add the hot horseradish sauce, to taste. Serve the paté on the thick slices of cucumber (or on seeded crackers – see page 75) or with vegetable batons as a dip.

- **CALORIES** 270
- PROTEIN 14G
- FAT 23G
- FIBRE 0G
- CARBS 3G

Guacamole

Perfect as a dip or as a side dish to add a bit of zing to a meal.

Makes 2 portions

1 ripe avocado, roughly mashed
½ chilli, deseeded and finely chopped (or chilli flakes to taste)
Juice of half a lime (or lemon)
2 large slices of beef tomato

Mash the avocado in a bowl with the chilli, lime juice and some seasoning. Spread the guacamole on a couple of slices of tomato, or serve it with vegetable batons as a dip.

- **CALORIES** 140
- PROTEIN 3G
- FAT 28G
- FIBRE 5G
- CARBS 5G

Why nuts make the ideal snack

For many years we've been wary of nuts because of their high fat and calorie content. Big mistake! Lots of studies have shown that eating a small handful of nuts a day actually helps you lose weight and cuts the risk of heart disease. Nuts are a key ingredient of the Mediterranean diet and, although it is true that they are fairly high in calories, your body finds them hard to digest and consequently many of those calories are not absorbed.

Packed with protein, fibre and healthy essential fats, they keep you full without significantly increasing your blood sugars, and contribute to the good bacteria in your gut, too. Go for salt-free nuts if you can, because you are less likely to overeat with them.

Savoury Brazil nut butter

Makes 4 portions

- CALORIES [illegible]
- PROTEIN [illegible]
- FAT [illegible]
- FIBRE [illegible]
- CARBS [illegible]

180g Brazil nuts, soaked in water for 24 hours, drained and rinsed
2–3 garlic cloves
3 tbsp lemon juice
4 tbsp rapeseed oil
2 tbsp tahini
Pinch of cayenne pepper

Blend all the ingredients in a food processor until you have a smooth paste. Loosen it with a little water if necessary and season it with a pinch of salt and black pepper. Transfer it to a bowl, cover it with clingfilm and chill it in the fridge until you want to use it. Serve it with batons of carrots, celery, peppers or cauliflower.

Healthy ploughman's

Cheese goes brilliantly with fruit such as apples or pears. It also works well with blackberries or blueberries. For a super-simple lunch snack, take a matchbox-sized piece of hard cheese, an apple or pear, or a handful of berries, along with a stick of celery and a couple of seeded crackers (see recipe below).

Thin seeded crackers

Perfect for eating with a dip or with cheese. These thin crackers contain lots of fibre and omega 3, and are an excellent source of heart-healthy, inflammation-reducing, essential fatty acids.

Makes 24 small crackers
(calories per cracker)

100ml water
60g spelt flour (or any wholegrain flour)
Extra flavouring, such as black pepper, chilli, rosemary or thyme
120g seeds made up of equal amounts of golden linseeds (or flax seeds), chia seeds, sunflower seeds and sesame seeds
¼ tsp Maldon salt
1 heaped tsp Marmite (or yeast extract equivalent – optional)

Preheat the oven to 150°C. In a medium-sized bowl, mix the flour and 50ml cold water. In a separate bowl, dissolve the Marmite in 50ml hot water and pour it into the flour. Add extra flavouring or herbs, if using. Now stir in the seeds and the Maldon salt. Leave the dough to bind for 15 minutes, stirring occasionally.

Line a large baking tray with baking paper and brush oil liberally over the surface or use a silicon baking tray. Tip the mixture onto the tray and spread it very thinly with the back of a fork, to about 3mm thick. Sprinkle over a little extra Maldon salt and bake it for about 20 minutes.

Then, using a knife, slice the cooked biscuit into small crackers. Carefully remove them from the baking paper and turn them over. Return them to the oven for 10-20 minutes or until they start to turn golden. Turn the oven off but leave them inside for a further 15-30 minutes to let them dry out. They can be stored in an airtight container for up to a week.

Tip: make sure chia makes up a quarter of the seed mixture, as it helps to bind the biscuits. The rest of the seeds can be adjusted according to taste.

- **CALORIES** 50
- PROTEIN 2G
- FAT 4G
- FIBRE 1G
- CARBS 2G

Seedy flapjacks

Made with wholesome, unprocessed nuts, seeds and fruit, and no added sugar, these seedy flapjacks have a deliciously chewy texture.

Makes 24 small squares
(calories per flapjack)

150g coconut oil
120g blueberries (or figs, chopped)
110g soft dates, finely chopped (about 15 large dates)
50g jumbo oats
100g rolled oats (ideally with bran)
3 tbsp mixed seeds (sunflower, pumpkin, sesame...)
3 tbsp hazelnuts (or almonds), roasted and chopped
3 tbsp dried cranberries (or goji berries or raisins)
Pinch of salt

Preheat the oven to 170°C and line a greased 20cm square metal baking tray with greaseproof paper. In a food processor, blitz the coconut oil, blueberries and dates. Mix in the oats, seeds, nuts, dried fruit and salt. Press the mixture down flat in the tray and bake it for about 30 minutes. Let the tray cool for about 10-20 minutes, and then cut the flapjacks into small squares before they set and carefully lay them out on a rack to dry. They can be stored in an airtight container for a few days.

- **CALORIES** 80
- PROTEIN 2G
- FAT 4G
- FIBRE 1G
- CARBS 10G

Parmesan crisps

A delicious and surprisingly healthy alternative to cheese straws. What's more, they take only 2 minutes to prepare and less than that to cook.

Makes 8 portions

100g Parmesan, finely grated
100g Cheddar, grated
100g ground almonds

Preheat the oven to 150°C and line a non-stick baking tray with greaseproof paper. Mix the cheeses and almonds together in a bowl, then, using a dessertspoon, drop dollops of the mixture on the tray. Cook them in the oven for 2 minutes, until they start to brown round the edges. Let them cool slightly and then tuck in.

Tip: to prevent the paper on the baking tray curling up at the edges, stick it in place with a few blobs of strategically placed oil.

- **CALORIES** 180
- PROTEIN 10G
- FAT 15G
- FIBRE 1G
- CARBS 1G

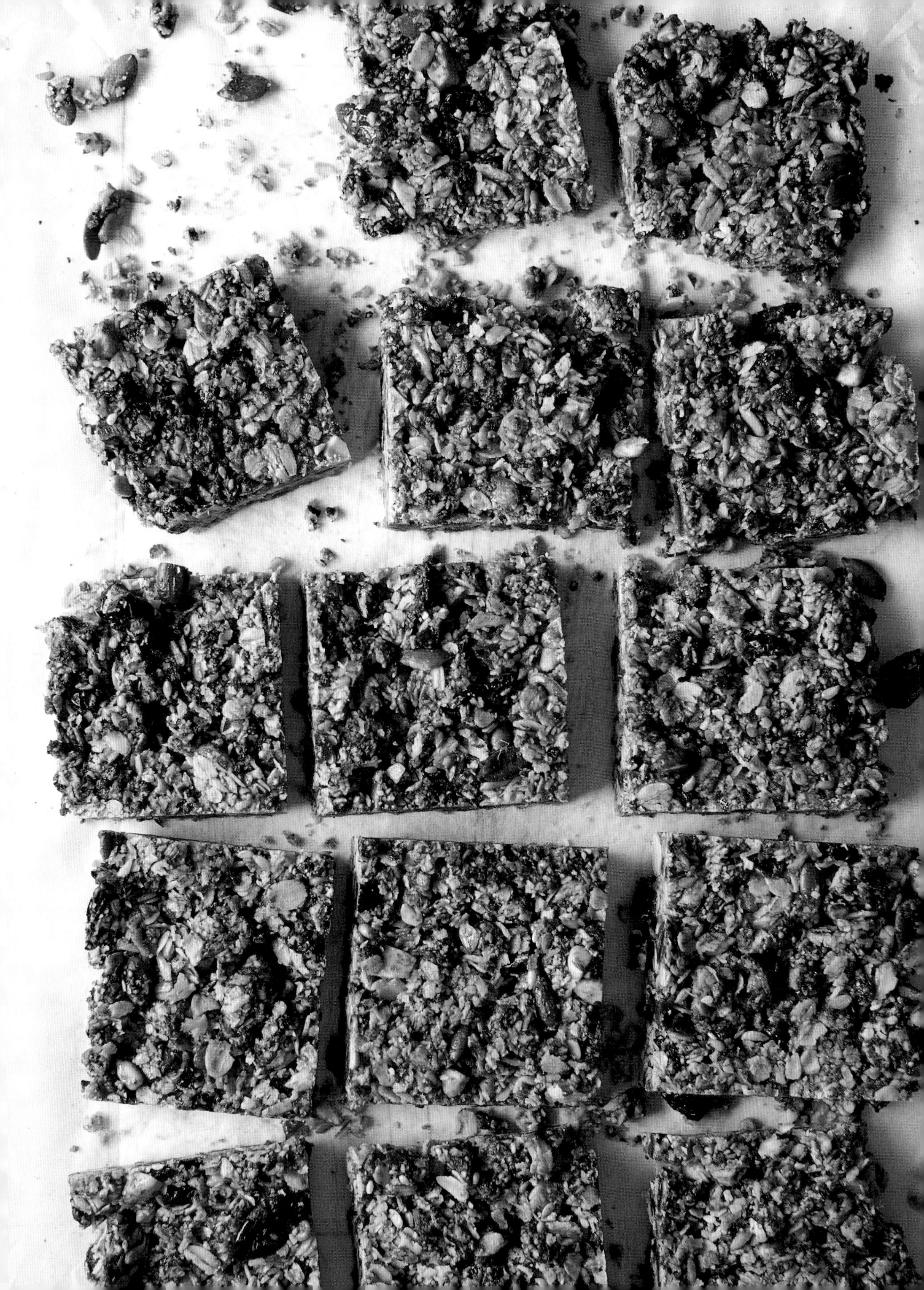

Easy Weekday Suppers

Simplicity and speed are the name of the game here. You will find many familiar favourites, lightly tweaked to replace starchy foods with delicious alternatives, and lots of other tasty and satisfying low-carb recipes that will help you lose weight and improve your blood sugars.

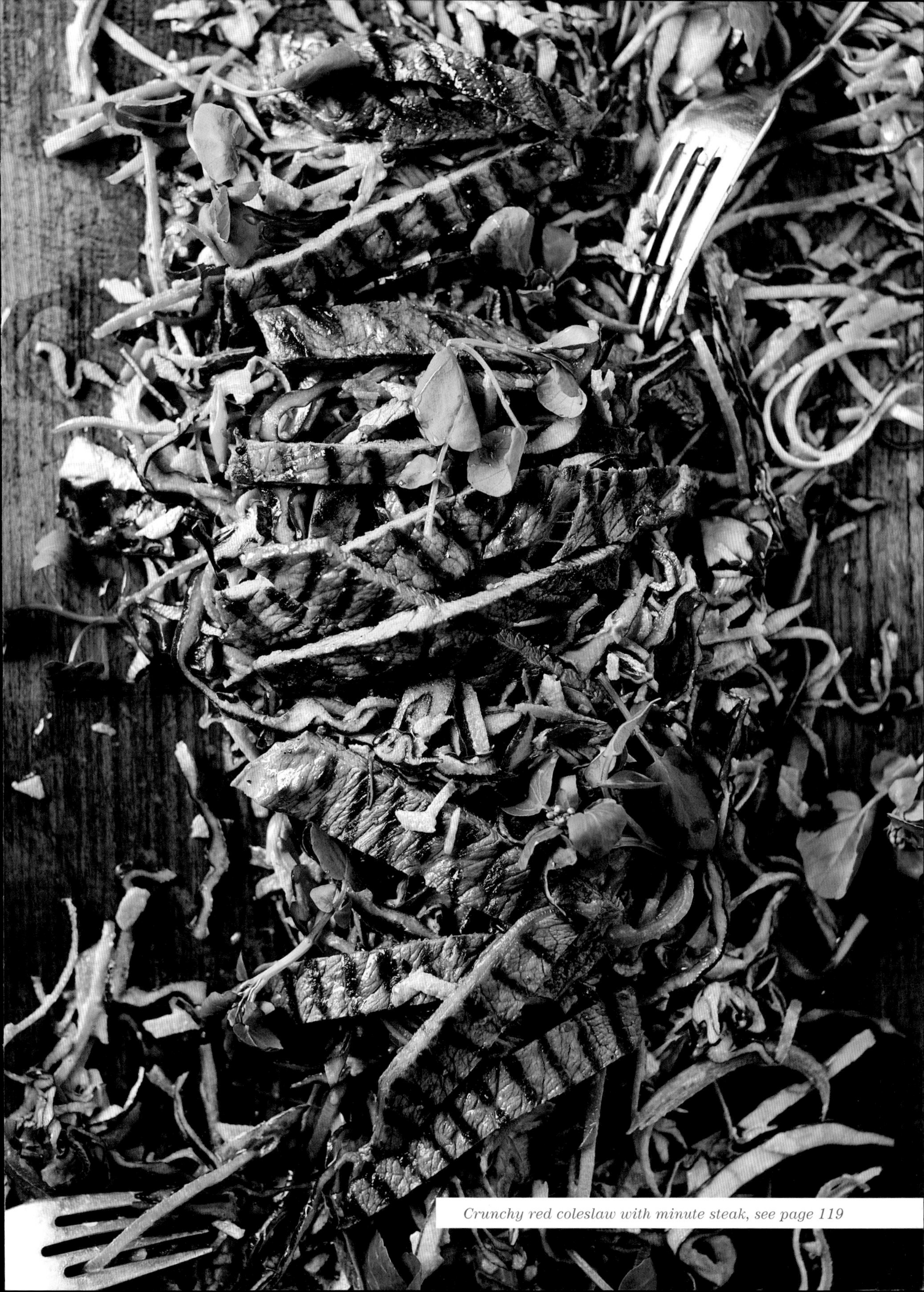

Crunchy red coleslaw with minute steak, see page 119

Roasted red pepper with anchovies

A scrumptious light supper, served here with quinoa or brown rice to mop up the juices.

Serves 1

1 red pepper
2-3 medium mushrooms, finely diced
1 tbsp pine nuts
6 cherry tomatoes, halved
1 tbsp olive oil
1 garlic clove, finely chopped or crushed
4 anchovies in oil
Handful of basil or coriander leaves

Preheat the oven to 200°C. Cut the red pepper in half, remove the stalk and seeds and place it in a baking dish. In a bowl, mix the diced mushrooms, pine nuts, garlic and tomatoes, along with most of the olive oil. Spoon the diced mushroom mixture into the pepper halves. Lay the anchovies on top, drizzle with the remaining olive oil and season with black pepper.

Bake the pepper in the oven for 20-25 minutes, or until some of the edges are slightly charred and the flesh has softened. Pour any juices in the dish over the pepper and garnish with basil or coriander. Serve with a salad of mixed leaves and rocket and 2 tbsp brown rice or quinoa (adds 35 calories).

- **CALORIES** 120
- PROTEIN 6G
- FAT 7G
- FIBRE 3G
- CARBS 10G

Spicy spinach and lentils

A wonderful filling dahl, full of rich creamy flavours and surprisingly filling.

Serves 2 as a main (or 4 as a side dish)

2 tbsp olive or coconut oil
1 small onion, chopped
2 garlic cloves, chopped
1-2 chillies, deseeded and finely diced (or 1-2 tsp dried chillies)
2 tsp cumin seeds
1 tsp ground coriander
1 tsp turmeric (optional)
2cm root ginger, diced
Juice of half a lemon
400ml tin coconut milk
200g green lentils, rinsed (or 400g tin green lentils, drained and rinsed)
200ml water if using dry lentils (just a dash if using tinned)
200g fresh or frozen spinach, defrosted
Handful of fresh coriander, chopped

In a medium-sized pan or casserole with a lid, gently fry the onion in the oil for 5-10 minutes. Stir in the garlic and cook for 1 more minute before adding the rest of the spices and the ginger. Cook for 2 minutes, then add the lemon juice, coconut milk and lentils. Cover and simmer for 20 minutes (or for 5 minutes if using tinned lentils), stirring occasionally and adding more water if needed. When the lentils are beginning to soften, tip in the spinach and cook for a further 3-5 minutes. Season and serve with fresh coriander stirred through.

Tip: to make the dish more substantial you can add a handful of roasted cashew nuts, fried chicken or paneer cheese; just adjust the calories accordingly.

- **CALORIES** 320
- PROTEIN 7G
- FAT 26G
- FIBRE 3G
- CARBS 14G

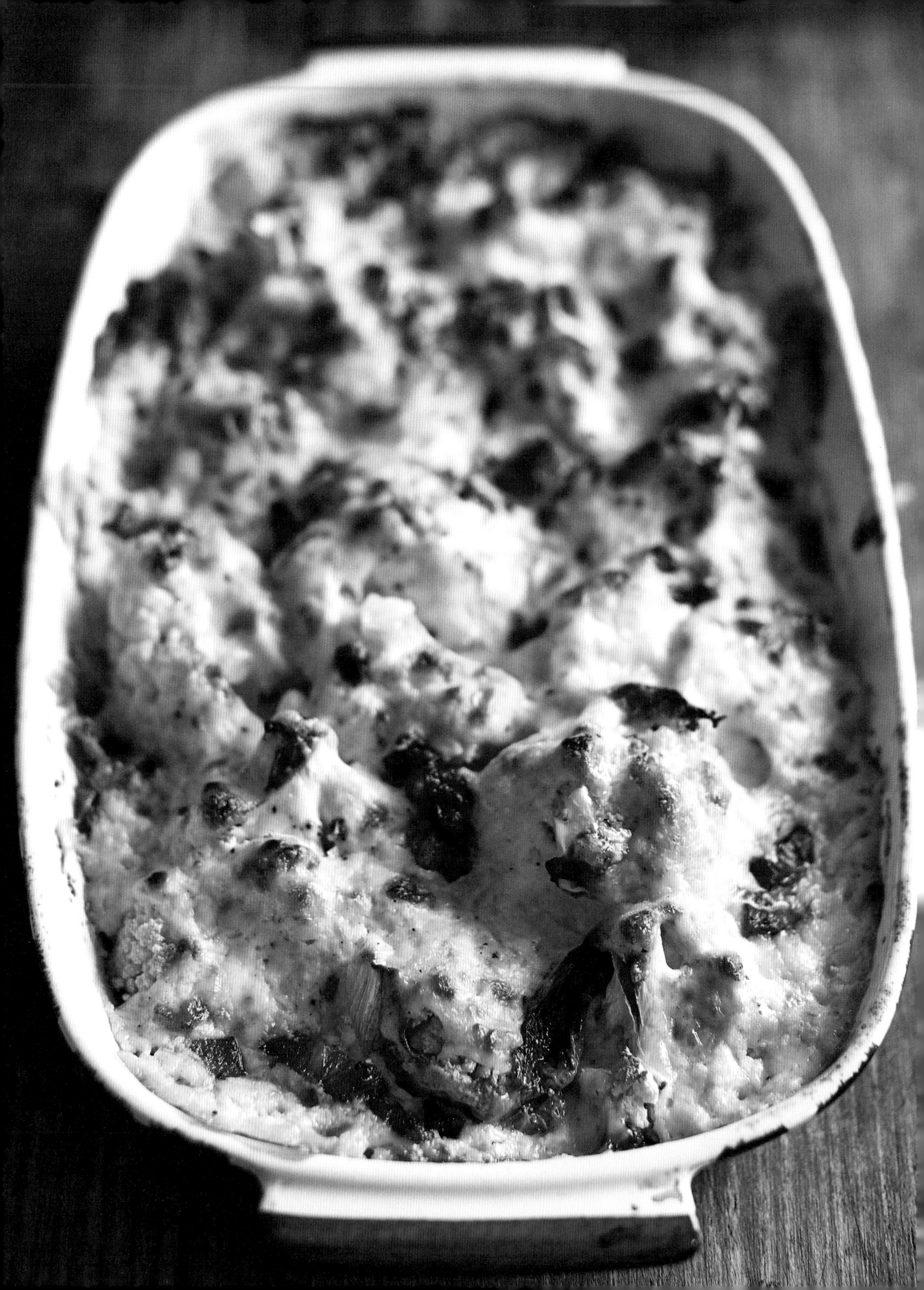

Cauliflower cheese

An old favourite with a low-carb, higher-fat twist. I enjoy munching jalapeños with mine, so have suggested mixing them in to give it a bit of a kick.

Serves 4

2 medium cauliflowers, broken into florets
200g ricotta
200ml crème fraîche
½ tbsp Worcestershire sauce
100g mature Cheddar, grated
50g diced bacon or lardons, fried (optional)
2-3 large jalapeño peppers from a jar, deseeded and finely diced (optional)
50g Parmesan, grated

Preheat the oven to 160°C. Place the cauliflower florets in a baking dish in the oven. In a medium-sized bowl, mix together the ricotta, crème fraîche, Worcestershire sauce and Cheddar and season with salt and freshly ground black pepper. Remove the cauliflower from the oven after about 5 minutes, stir in the bacon and jalapeño peppers, if using, then pour over the cheese sauce. Scatter the Parmesan over the surface and return the dish to the oven for 20-30 minutes, or until the mixture is bubbling and brown on top. Serve with fresh greens.

Tip: substitute some of the cauliflower with broccoli to give the dish more colour.

- **CALORIES** 450
- PROTEIN 20G
- FAT 39G
- FIBRE 2G
- CARBS 5G

Cajun-spiced bean burgers

These tasty bean burgers offer the rich heat of the deep south.

Serves 4

200g celeriac, peeled and diced
3 tbsp olive oil
1 small onion, finely diced
2 garlic cloves, finely chopped
1-2 red chillies, deseeded and finely diced
2 tsp Cajun spice (or see tips)
400g tin mixed beans, drained and rinsed
Small bunch of coriander, chopped
2 eggs, beaten
40g pine nuts, chopped
2 tsp chia seeds
1 lime, quartered
Handful of rocket leaves

Preheat the oven to 200°C. Place the celeriac in a pan of boiling water and cook it for 8-10 minutes or until it is tender, then drain it and set it aside. Heat 1 tbsp olive oil in a small frying pan, and fry the onion, garlic, chilli and Cajun spice for 2-3 minutes.

Transfer the mixture to a bowl, stir in the beans, celeriac and coriander, season well and mash energetically to bind everything together. Leave the mixture to cool slightly, then add the eggs, pine nuts and chia seeds. Mix well to combine. With wet hands, divide the mixture into 4 and shape it into patties. Put them in the fridge to chill for 30 minutes.

Drizzle 1 tbsp oil on a non-stick baking tray, place the patties on it and bake them for about 25 minutes, checking after about 15 minutes and drizzling on a bit more oil so they don't dry out. Serve on a bed of rocket leaves with a wedge of lime, and perhaps some guacamole (see page 73), and a dollop of soured cream (add 30 calories).

Tips: you can make your own Cajun spice by combining ½ tsp each of dried oregano, paprika, cayenne pepper (or chilli flakes) and black pepper, along with ¼ tsp salt. Extra burgers can be frozen, uncooked. Bake them from frozen for 40-45 minutes.

- **CALORIES** 300
- PROTEIN 13G
- FAT 20G
- FIBRE 1G
- CARBS 20G

Turkey burgers

Serves 6

500g minced turkey (or lean pork)
4 spring onions or 1 leek, finely diced
4 fresh or soft dried apricots, very finely chopped
100g halloumi, finely diced (or 100g chopped cashews)
1 egg, beaten
Handful of coriander, finely chopped
½ tsp chilli flakes, to taste
1 tbsp olive oil

Mash all the ingredients except the olive oil together in a bowl so the flavours meld and season with salt and black pepper. Shape the mixture into 6 balls and place them on a plate. Flatten them slightly, then leave them in the fridge for half an hour to firm up. Heat the olive oil in a frying pan and gently fry the burgers on both sides until they are cooked through. Serve with salad (they go well with crunchy red coleslaw, see page 119) and 2 tbsp quinoa or bulgar wheat (add 35 calories).

Tip: these are also delicious as nibbles if you make them into smaller, bite-sized balls and serve them with a tasty dip such as tzatziki (see page 72).

- **CALORIES** 180
- PROTEIN 26G
- FAT 8G
- FIBRE 1G
- CARBS 2G

Chinese pork meatballs

Serves 6

500g pork mince
2 eggs, beaten
4 spring onions, finely chopped
2 garlic cloves, finely chopped (or 2 tsp garlic paste)
½ tsp chilli flakes
½ tsp Chinese 5 spice
1 tbsp Thai fish sauce
2 tbsp sesame oil
2 tbsp coriander, finely chopped

Preheat the oven to 180°C (if baking, rather than frying; see below). Mix all the ingredients together thoroughly in a bowl, then roll the mixture into balls about the size of a plum. Either bake them on a greased baking sheet for 15-20 minutes or fry them gently in a pan. Serve with 600g stir-fried Swiss chard (see page 168). You could also add a portion of konjac noodles (see page 198).

- **CALORIES** 160
- PROTEIN 21G
- FAT 8G
- FIBRE 1G
- CARBS 1G

Quick quiche in a dish

This no-pastry quiche was suggested by a great friend, Nicola, who sent me the recipe as a short text. It sounded too easy to be true, but it really is as simple as it is delicious.

Serves 4

4 eggs
100ml crème fraîche
100g strong Cheddar, grated
2 spring onions, diced
5 balls of frozen spinach, defrosted and drained
½ tsp ground nutmeg

Preheat the oven to 170°C and lightly grease either an ovenproof dish or separate ramekins. With a fork whisk together the eggs and crème fraîche, then stir in the rest of the ingredients with some seasoning. Pour the mixture into the dish(es) and bake it in the oven for about 25 minutes (10 minutes less if using ramekins).

- **CALORIES** 280
- PROTEIN 16G
- FAT 24G
- FIBRE 2G
- CARBS 1G

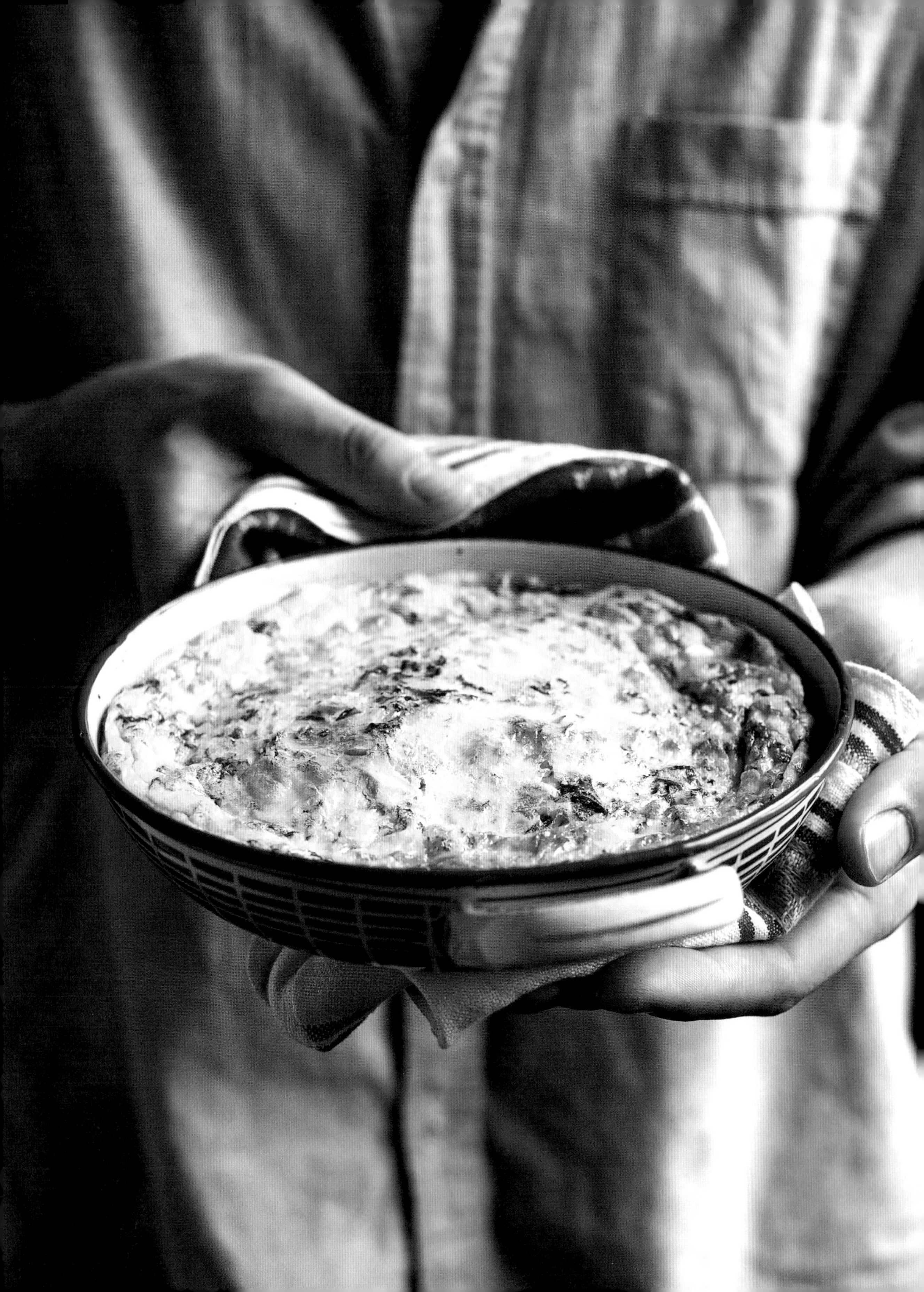

Chicken drumsticks 2 ways

1. Lightly chillied

No starchy batter or breadcrumbs here. Instead, the drumsticks are lightly crusted with ground almonds, salt, pepper and a hint of chilli.

Serves 4

50g ground almonds
50g Parmesan, grated
2 tbsp full-fat mayonnaise
2 tbsp light olive oil
1 tbsp sweet chilli sauce (from a jar, or ideally make your own, see page 175)
8 chicken drumsticks

Preheat the oven to 180°C. Mix the almonds and Parmesan in a bowl and season well with salt and plenty of freshly ground black pepper. Mix the mayonnaise in a separate bowl with most of the olive oil and the sweet chilli sauce. Coat the chicken in this mixture, then roll it in the almond and Parmesan mixture. Put it in the fridge for 10-15 minutes to allow the crust to firm up, then place it on a greased roasting tray and drizzle the remaining olive oil over it. Bake it for 20-25 minutes, or until the juices run clear (not pink) when pierced with a sharp knife. Serve with a salad or steamed greens.

- **CALORIES** 410
- PROTEIN 31G
- FAT 30G
- FIBRE 1G
- CARBS 4G

---

2. With a garlic crust

Serves 4

50g ground almonds
50g Parmesan, grated
2 tbsp full-fat mayonnaise
2 tbsp light olive oil
2 tbsp Dijon mustard
2 garlic cloves, crushed
8 chicken drumsticks

Preheat the oven to 180°C. Mix the Parmesan and almonds in a bowl and season well with salt and plenty of freshly ground black pepper. Mix together the mayonnaise, 1 tbsp olive oil, mustard and garlic in a separate bowl. Coat the chicken in this mixture, then roll it in the almond and Parmesan mixture. Put it in the fridge for 10-15 minutes to allow the crust to firm up, then place it on a greased roasting tray and drizzle the remaining olive oil over it. Bake it for 20-25 minutes, or until the juices run clear (not pink) when pierced with a sharp knife. Serve with a salad or steamed greens.

- **CALORIES** 440
- PROTEIN 33G
- FAT 34G
- FIBRE 2G
- CARBS 2G

Chicken wrapped in Parma ham

The chicken absorbs the flavours from the Parma ham which forms a delicious crust around it.

Serves 2

1 heaped tbsp full-fat cream cheese
1 garlic clove, crushed or finely chopped (or use ready-made garlic cream cheese)
2 small skinless chicken breasts
6 slices of Parma ham (or a cheaper equivalent such as prosciutto or serrano)
1 tbsp olive oil

Preheat the oven to 180°C. Mix together the cream cheese and garlic and season with black pepper and a pinch of salt. Spread the mixture over the surface of the chicken breasts and wrap 2-3 slices of ham around each one. Drizzle the olive oil over the chicken, place it in an oven dish and bake it for 20-25 minutes, or until the juices run clear (not pink) when pierced with a sharp knife. Serve with a salad or green vegetables.

- **CALORIES** 320
- PROTEIN 39G
- FAT 18G
- FIBRE 0G
- CARBS 0G

Spicy tuna fish patties

This is a bit like a tuna falafel and was inspired by a recipe by Stacey on the Blood Sugar Diet website. Wonderfully quick and easy to whizz together.

Serves 4

2 x 185g tins tuna in olive oil, drained
400g tin chickpeas, drained and rinsed
3 spring onions, diced
½ red pepper, deseeded and diced
1-2 red chillies, deseeded and finely diced (or 1-2 tsp chilli paste or flakes)
2 eggs
½ tsp ground cumin
2 tbsp olive oil
Juice of 2 limes
Handful of coriander or parsley, chopped (optional)
8 small cocktail gherkins (around 50g), finely diced

Mix the tuna, chickpeas, spring onions, red pepper, chillies, eggs and cumin together with 1 tbsp olive oil and the juice of 1 lime in a bowl. Pulse for a few seconds with a hand blender or a food processor, stir and pulse again for a few more seconds. This mixture should still have some texture. Then add the coriander and diced gherkins and mix them in thoroughly.

Divide the mixture into 8, shaping them into patties. Place them in the fridge for half an hour to firm up. Then heat the rest of the olive oil in a large frying pan and fry them 4 at a time. When the egg has set enough for them to be turned without crumbling, flip them over. Squeeze the juice of the second lime over the patties just before serving along with tzatziki (see page 72) and a light salad or fresh greens.

Tip: if the mixture seems a bit runny, add 1-2 tsp chia seeds to bind it.

- **CALORIES** 310
- PROTEIN 31G
- FAT 17G
- FIBRE 3G
- CARBS 11G

Indian-spiced prawns

A deliciously light, tangy prawn curry. Adapted from a recipe from the mother of my friend and colleague Durgesh.

Serves 2

250g large raw prawns (or frozen cooked prawns, defrosted)
¼ tsp chilli powder (to taste)
¼ tsp turmeric
1 tsp tamarind paste (or ½ tbsp mirin or juice of half a lime)
1 tbsp vegetable oil
1 large onion, finely chopped
2 garlic cloves, crushed or finely chopped
1 cinnamon stick, broken in two
½ 400g tin chopped tomatoes
100g spinach (frozen or fresh)

Marinate the prawns in the chilli powder, turmeric and tamarind paste for 30 minutes. Meanwhile, heat the oil in a non-stick saucepan and sauté the onions until they start to turn golden brown, then add the garlic and cinnamon stick. After 2-3 minutes, add the tomatoes and the marinade (not the prawns). Check the seasoning and cook the sauce on a moderate heat until it starts to thicken. Then turn the heat to low and stir in the prawns and spinach. Cook the prawns until they change colour if using fresh (about 10 minutes) or for about 5 minutes if they are already cooked, stirring occasionally. Serve with cauliflower rice (see page 98) or stir-fried cabbage (see page 169).

- **CALORIES** 190
- PROTEIN 24G
- FAT 7G
- FIBRE 2G
- CARBS 10G

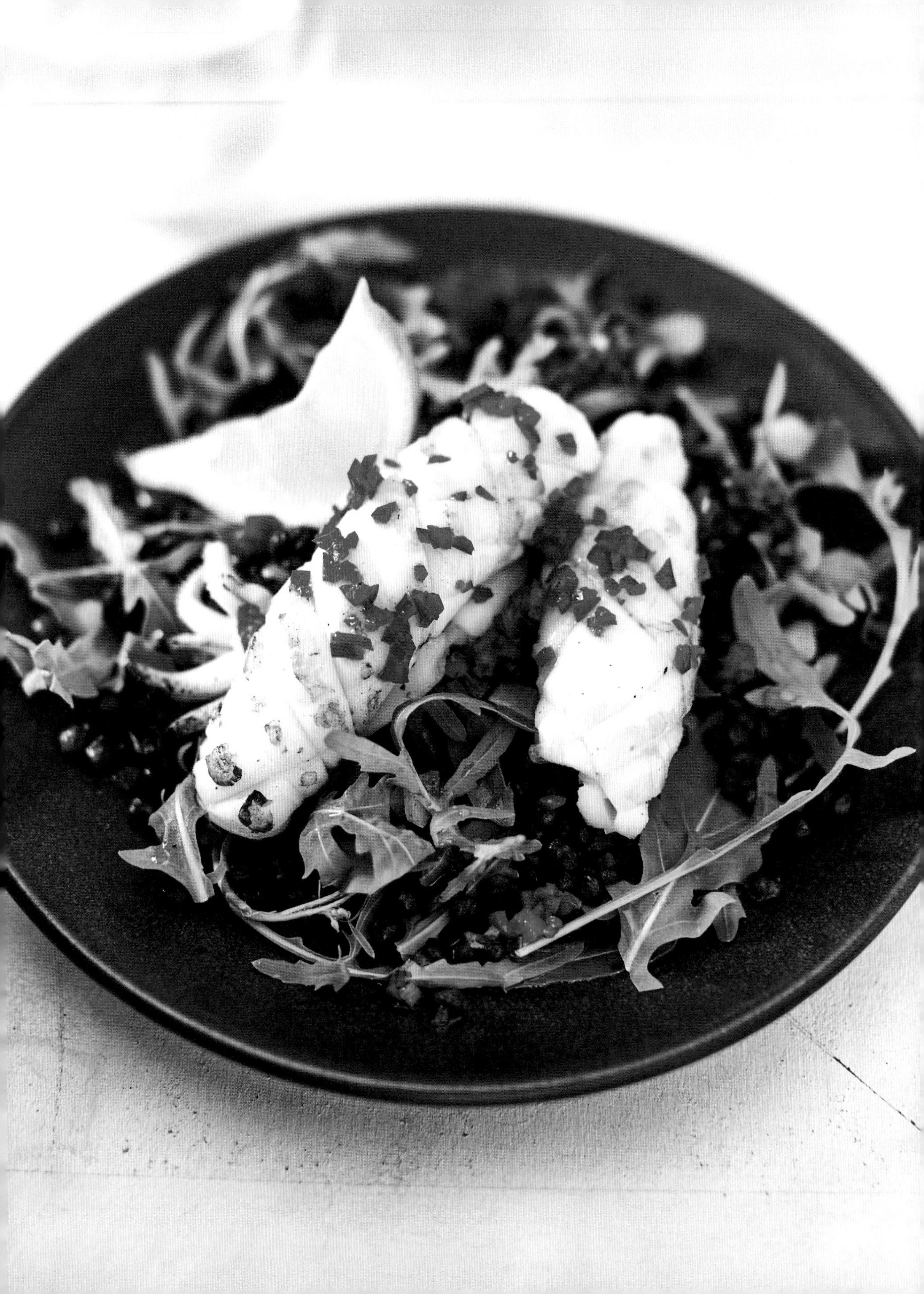

Chilli squid with lentils

The chilli enhances the flavours of the squid here beautifully.

Serves 4

1 tbsp olive oil
1 small onion, diced
250g pack ready-cooked Puy lentils (or cook from scratch)
Juice of half a lemon
4 medium-sized squid, cleaned
4 generous tsp sweet chilli sauce (see page 175; or 3 large red chillies, diced and mixed with 2 tbsp extra-virgin olive oil and seasoned)

Prepare the lentils first. Sweat the onion in olive oil until it starts to brown. Stir in the lentils and simmer for a few minutes to heat them through. Season with salt and black pepper and the lemon juice.

Cut each squid tube open, lay it flat and score the inner surface with a sharp knife in cross-hatch lines about 1cm apart. Season them and cook them on a very hot griddle with the cross-hatched side down for 1-2 minutes, then turn them over – they will curl up almost immediately, indicating that they are cooked.

To serve, place the lentils on the plates with the squid on top, each with a generous tsp of chilli sauce. This dish goes well with a rocket salad, drizzled with olive oil and lemon juice.

Tip: home-cooked Puy lentils taste even better, with a slightly stronger peppery flavour.

- **CALORIES** 160
- PROTEIN 18G
- FAT 5G
- FIBRE 3G
- CARBS 13G

Salmon 3 ways

1. With lemon and dill nut crust on roasted veg

Serves 4

3 peppers, preferably red and yellow, chopped into large pieces
2 courgettes, roughly sliced
2 red onions, chopped into wedges
Drizzle of olive oil
1 small egg
Zest of 1 lemon
Handful of dill, finely chopped
1 tbsp walnuts, crushed
2 tbsp ground almonds
4 salmon fillets

Preheat the oven to 180°C. Put the peppers, courgettes and onions in a baking dish or tray, season them and drizzle the olive oil over. Start baking them in the oven while you prepare the fish. Beat the egg in a bowl and add the lemon zest, dill, walnuts and ground almonds and mix well. Season with a pinch of salt and plenty of black pepper.

Remove the vegetables from the oven after 10 minutes and place the salmon on top, leaving a gap between each fillet. Spoon the nut crumb mixture evenly over each fillet and return them to the oven for another 15-20 minutes (be careful not to overcook them as they will dry out).

- **CALORIES** 370
- PROTEIN 28G
- FAT 23G
- FIBRE 4G
- CARBS 14G

---

2. With coconut and chilli

A fabulous and easy Indian recipe by our good friends, Drs Rajsingh and Rai.

Serves 1

1 salmon fillet
1 tsp lemon juice
1 tsp light olive oil
1 small onion, diced
2cm root ginger, grated
2 garlic cloves, finely chopped
1-2 green chillies, deseeded and diced (to taste)
Handful of coriander, roughly chopped
1 tbsp fresh coconut, grated (or ½ tbsp desiccated coconut)

Preheat the oven to 180°C. Season the fish, then drizzle over the lemon juice and leave it to marinate for 30-60 minutes. Heat the oil in a small frying pan and sauté the onion until it is soft – about 5 minutes. Add the ginger, garlic, chillies and coriander and continue to cook gently on a medium heat for 2-3 minutes before adding the grated coconut and salt to taste. Stir for another minute, then remove the pan from the heat. Place the fish on a baking tray and spread the mixture over it. Bake it for about 20 minutes. Serve with steamed green veg such as mange tout or fine beans.

Tip: fresh grated coconut can be kept in the freezer.

- **CALORIES** 300
- PROTEIN 22G
- FAT 20G
- FIBRE 3G
- CARBS 7G

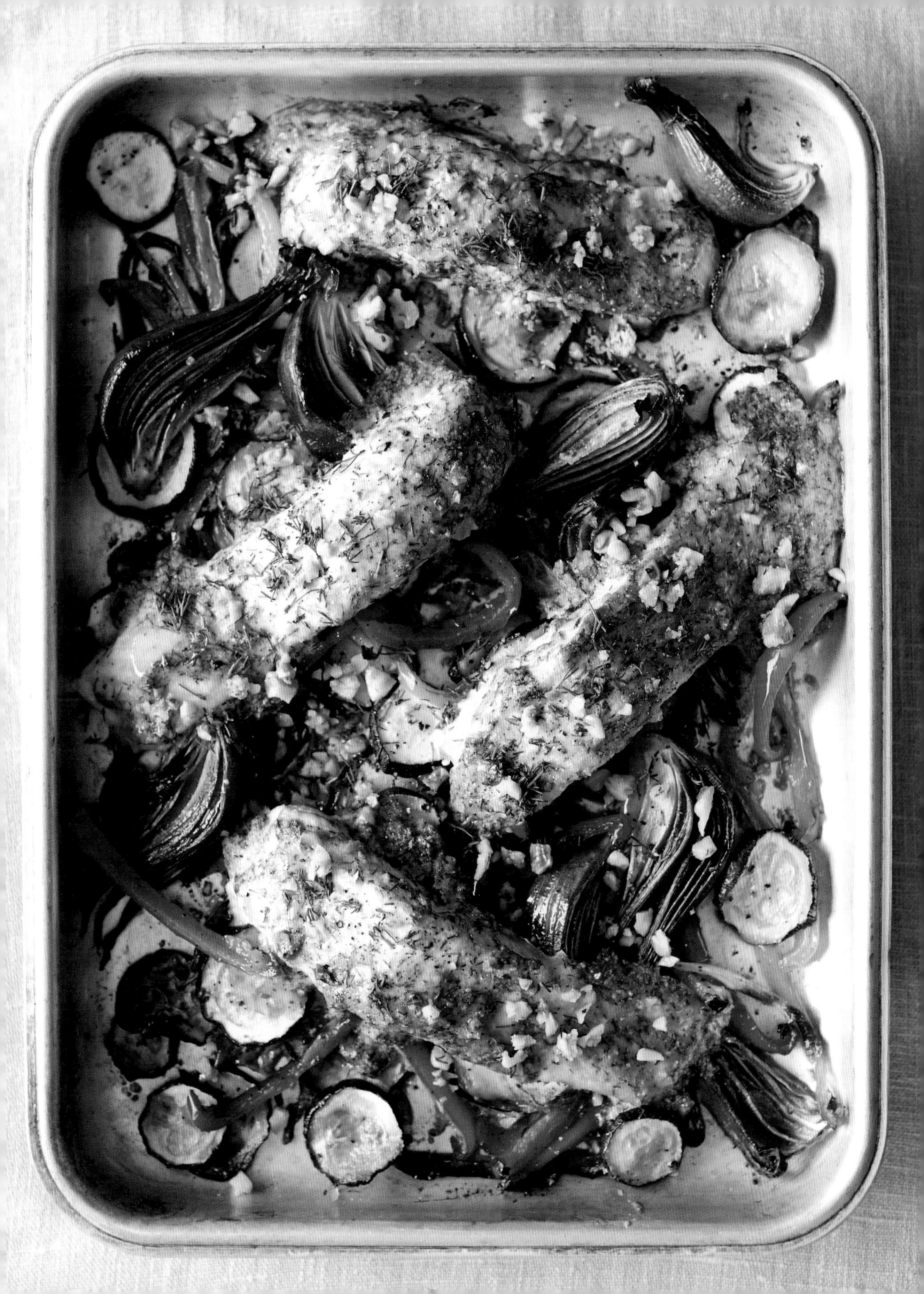

3. With ginger

This is an old favourite of ours. Purists may prefer to swap the ginger in syrup for a knob of fresh ginger, but the tiny amount of extra sugar eaten with the meal is insignificant.

Serves 6

6 medium-sized salmon fillets
2 tbsp Thai fish sauce
2 red peppers, deseeded and cut into strips
3 spring onions, sliced lengthwise
Juice of 1 medium orange
1 knob of ginger in syrup, drained and finely diced
1 red chilli, deseeded and finely chopped
½ tbsp olive oil
Handful of coriander or parsley, chopped

Preheat the oven to 180°C. Place the salmon in a shallow baking dish to marinate in the Thai fish sauce for 10-20 minutes. Scatter the spring onions and red pepper strips around the salmon pieces, then pour over the orange juice. Sprinkle the ginger and chilli on top. Drizzle with the olive oil and season well. Bake the salmon in the oven for about 20 minutes. Sprinkle over the coriander and serve with green vegetables such as kale or spring greens.

- CALORIES 210
- PROTEIN 21G
- FAT 11G
- FIBRE 1G
- CARBS 5G

Creamy skinny kedgeree

Serves 2

2 eggs
150ml semi-skimmed milk
2 bay leaves
180g smoked white fish, such as haddock
½ large cauliflower, grated
2 small onions, one diced, one cut finely into rings
2 tbsp coconut oil (or 40g butter)
2 tsp medium curry powder (1 tsp if using hot variety)
40g cooked peas (optional)
Squeeze of lemon (to taste)
Handful of parsley, chopped

Boil the eggs for 6-7 minutes, then plunge them into cold water to cool them before peeling them and cutting them in half. Meanwhile, pour the milk into a small saucepan with a lid. Add the bay leaves and fish (this can be cut up if necessary so that it lies flat) and simmer for 10 minutes. Remove the fish to a plate, keeping the milk in the pan. Allow the fish to cool a bit before removing the skin and flaking the flesh. Add the grated cauliflower to the milk and simmer for 5-7 minutes. Drain the milk into a bowl and put the cauliflower aside.

In a large frying pan, sweat the diced onion in 1 tbsp coconut oil for 5 minutes. Stir in the curry powder and cook gently for another 2-3 minutes. Then fold in the cauliflower 'rice', the flaked fish and the peas, if using, with enough of the infused milk to loosen the mixture. Simmer gently for a few minutes. Pour in extra milk if it seems to be drying out.

While the 'rice' cooks, in a separate pan, fry the onion rings in the rest of the oil until they are golden brown and slightly crispy. Add a squeeze of lemon to the kedgeree and serve it with the eggs on top, the onion rings and parsley scattered over, along with a grinding of black pepper.

- **CALORIES** 390
- PROTEIN 30G
- FAT 24G
- FIBRE 3G
- CARBS 12G

Rice swaps

Unfortunately, white rice is high in starch and rapidly leads to a spike in blood sugar in most people. Brown rice is better, but should still be eaten only occasionally. You can reduce the impact of eating brown rice on your blood sugar levels by adding 1-2 teaspoons of oil to the boiling water during cooking and then leaving it in the fridge for 12 hours (30g brown rice = 130 calories). Cooking and then cooling rice converts the carbohydrate in it into 'resistant' starch, a form which is more like fibre, and therefore has a lower GI. As brown rice takes longer to cook than white rice, we recommend keeping pre-prepared portions in the freezer. Not only will it be ready almost instantly when needed, but some of it will have become resistant starch in the process. Win win.

Cauliflower rice

This is a surprisingly good, low-carb replacement for rice. High in fibre and nutrients, cauliflower contains astonishingly few calories and has a very low GI. It has become so popular that supermarkets are selling it in their freezer section. If you are preparing your own, first grate your cauliflower (or blitz it in a food processor). Then there are various ways of cooking it (1 medium cauliflower makes 4 servings of 30 calories each):

BAKED: mix it with 1 tsp olive oil in a bowl then bake it in a medium oven for about 10 minutes – it will need occasional shaking and turning (add 30 calories per portion).

MICROWAVED: in a covered bowl for a minute or two until it's al dente and still slightly chewy.

STEAMED: for 5-7 minutes.

FRIED: simply fry it in 1 tbsp olive oil for 7-8 minutes until it's al dente (add 30 calories per portion).

Konjac rice

This is sold as 'low-carb rice' in pre-cooked packets. It is made of konjac glucomannan, a natural soluble fibre, and, like konjac noodle products, is very low in starchy carbohydrates and gluten-free. Konjac rice has a slightly rubbery texture and is best rinsed before use. It has no particular flavour of its own and works well when mixed with strong flavours such as in stir-fries, oriental salads or soups.

Quinoa

This has become an incredibly popular replacement for grains. If, like me, you are struggling with the pronunciation – it is pronounced 'keen-wah'. Like buckwheat, it is a pseudo-cereal and has a slightly nutty taste and chewy texture. Quinoa has significantly higher levels of protein, nutrients and fibre than rice and much less impact on blood sugars. But it is starchy, like brown rice, so eat it in moderation, 1-2 tbsp per serving. We particularly recommend the darker brown and red varieties, as these have a higher fibre content and more taste. It is very easy to cook.

Serves 2

60g quinoa
300ml chicken or vegetable stock

In a small saucepan, cover the quinoa with about 1-2cm stock and bring it to the boil. Put the lid on and turn down the heat to a gentle simmer for 10 minutes or until the water is absorbed. Then turn off the heat and leave it to steam with the lid on for a further 10 minutes.

- CALORIES 120
- PROTEIN 6G
- FAT 2G
- FIBRE 2G
- CARBS 22G

Bulgar wheat

Although bulgar wheat is not as high in protein or as low-carb as quinoa, it does have a fairly high fibre content.

Serves 2

80g bulgar wheat
200-300ml chicken or vegetable stock

In a small saucepan, cover the bulgar with about 1-2cm stock and bring it to the boil. Put the lid on and turn down the heat to a gentle simmer for 10 minutes. Then turn off the heat and leave it to steam with the lid on for a further 10 minutes.

- CALORIES 140
- PROTEIN 4G
- FAT 1G
- FIBRE 3G
- CARBS 31G

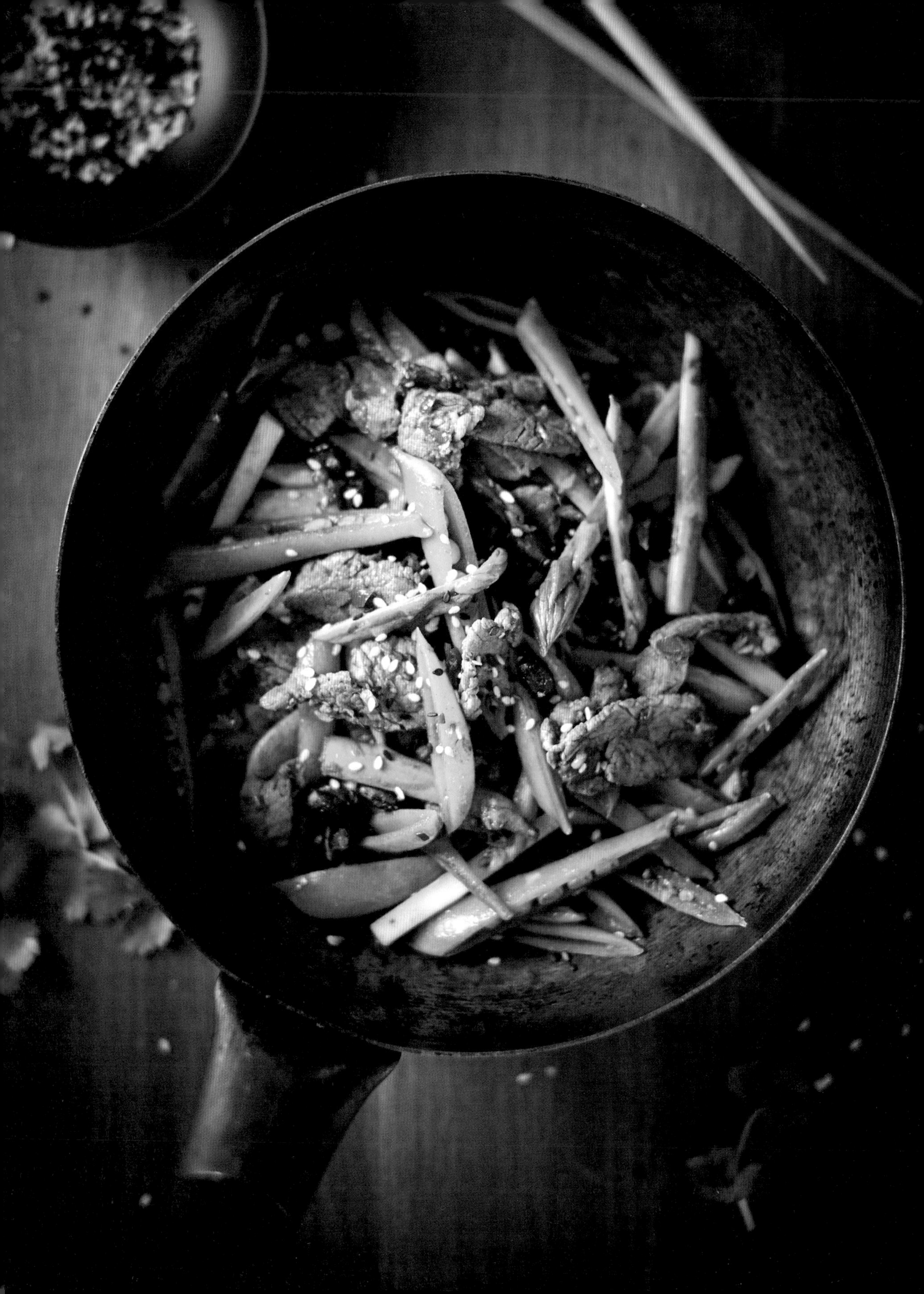

Beef stir-fry with asparagus and sesame seeds

We include asparagus here mainly because it tastes so delicious and complements the flavours. However, it also happens to contain plenty of inulin, which acts as a prebiotic, boosting the beneficial bacteria in the gut, and thereby helping to keep weight off and your blood sugars down.

Serves 2

200g beef fillet, thinly sliced
1 tbsp mirin (or sherry)
2 tbsp soy sauce
2cm root ginger, grated
1 garlic clove, finely chopped
1 red chilli, deseeded and finely diced (or 1 tsp chilli flakes)
½ 400g tin black beans
1 tbsp coconut or rapeseed oil
150g asparagus, cut into 3cm batons (if thick, slice the stalks lengthways too)
100g mange tout or sugar snap peas, chopped into thin sticks (optional)
1 tsp sesame oil (optional)
2 tsp sesame seeds
Handful of coriander leaves, torn

Mix together the mirin, ½ tbsp soy sauce, ginger, garlic and chilli in a bowl and marinate the beef fillet in it for 30 minutes. In a separate small bowl, marinate the black beans in ½ tbsp soy sauce. Place a wok over a high heat, add the oil, and then the beef mixture. Stir-fry for about 2 minutes, or until the meat is browned all over. Add the asparagus, mange tout, if using, black beans and sesame oil and reduce the heat. Then stir in 2 tbsp hot water and the remaining soy sauce and stir-fry gently for another minute or two, until the vegetables are just tender. Season with freshly ground black pepper and sprinkle over the sesame seeds and coriander leaves. Serve with cauliflower rice (see page 98).

- **CALORIES** 250
- PROTEIN 27G
- FAT 13G
- FIBRE 3G
- CARBS 5G

Chickpeas 2 ways

Chickpeas, one of the pulses recommended as part of a healthy Mediterranean-style diet, are quite high in protein, nutrients and fibre. They are also fairly high in carbohydrate, but when combined with vegetables and healthy oils the carbs are released relatively slowly, providing energy without significantly spiking blood sugars.

1. With Indian-spiced stir-fried greens

A delicious, quick meal that also works well as a side dish.

Serves 2

1 tbsp coconut or rapeseed oil
1 tsp mustard seeds
1 large onion, diced fairly small
5-6 curry leaves
2 green chillies, deseeded and diced, or 2 tsp chilli flakes (to taste)
½ tsp turmeric
½ 400g tin white lentils
½ 400g tin chickpeas
500g green cabbage, thinly sliced
1 tsp garam masala

Heat the oil in a large non-stick, wok-style pan. Add the mustard seeds and then the onions, curry leaves and green chillies. Sauté for 3-4 minutes on a low heat. Stir in the turmeric, lentils, chickpeas and cabbage. Season with salt, and cook on a high heat for 5-7 minutes, stirring constantly. Finally, mix in the garam masala and season to taste.

Tip: you can use dried chickpeas and lentils and boil them (separately) until they are al dente. Use about 120g of each, cooked and drained.

- **CALORIES** 390
- PROTEIN 22G
- FAT 13G
- FIBRE 18G
- CARBS 51G

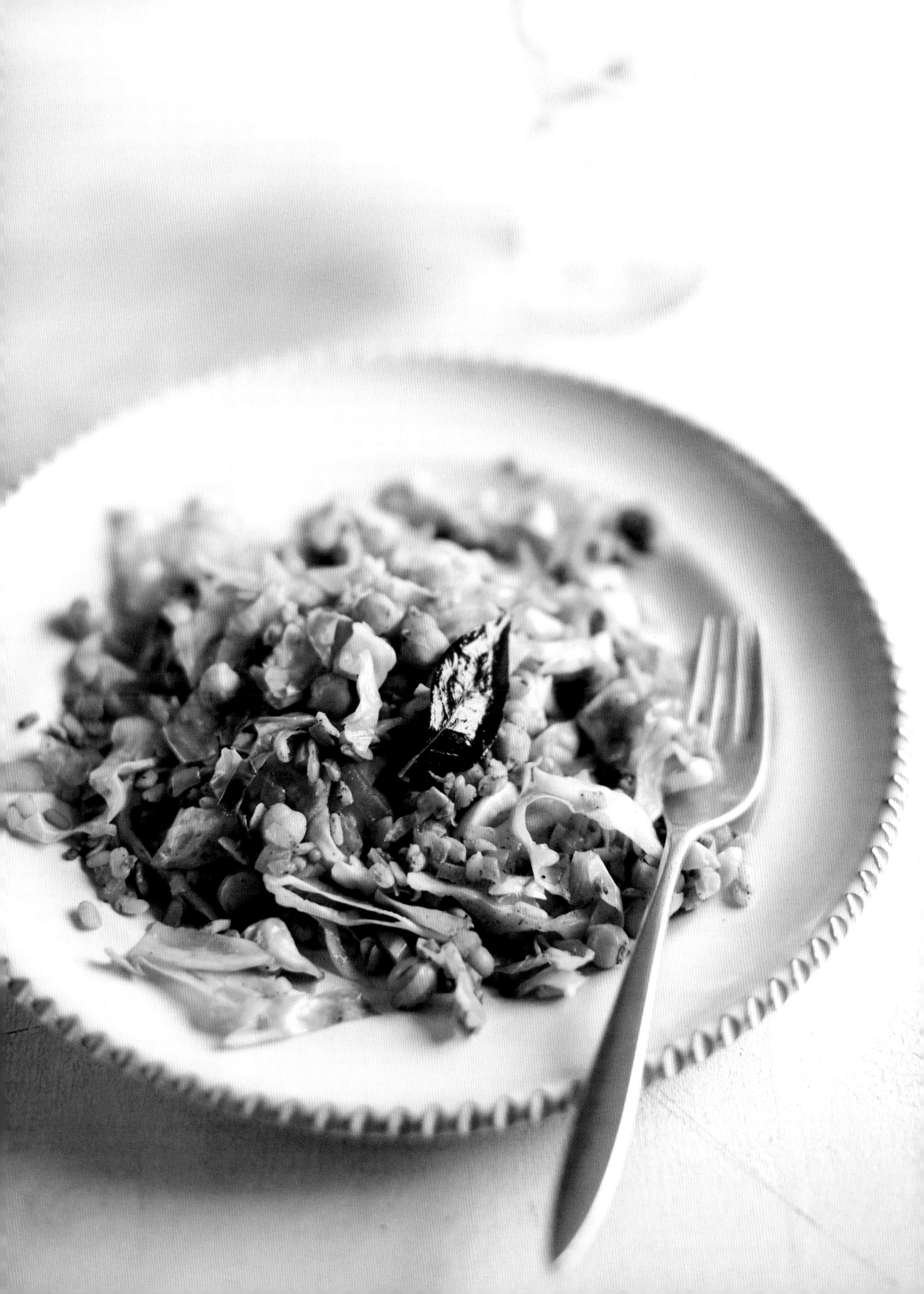

2. Chickpea chilli

A rich, vegetarian dish, super-easy to make.

Serves 2

1 medium onion, diced
2 tbsp olive oil
1 tsp ground cumin
½ tsp dried oregano
1 carrot, diced
1 red pepper, deseeded and diced
2 celery stalks, diced
100g mushrooms, chopped
1 garlic clove, diced or crushed
1 green chilli, deseeded and diced (more if you like it hot, or 1 tsp chilli paste or flakes)
400g tin chopped tomatoes
½ tbsp balsamic vinegar
400g tin chickpeas
½ 400g tin black beans (or kidney beans)
Handful of coriander leaves, chopped

Heat the oil in a large saucepan and sweat the onion for 5 minutes. Add the cumin and oregano, then the carrot, pepper, celery and mushrooms, and cook for a further 10 minutes. Stir in the garlic, chilli, tomatoes, vinegar, chickpeas and black beans, and simmer vigorously until the sauce has begun to reduce, about 10 minutes. Season to taste and serve with a scattering of coriander and a spoonful of raitha (see page 72).

Tips: this recipe works well with other types of beans. You could also include diced aubergine or courgette. It's very flexible.

- **CALORIES** 270
- PROTEIN 13G
- FAT 9G
- FIBRE 10G
- CARBS 36G

Stir-fried cabbage with peppered mackerel

So simple and delicious. I could live on this.

Serves 2

1 small onion, sliced
1 garlic clove, chopped
300g cabbage or spring greens, finely sliced
1 tbsp olive oil
2 peppered smoked mackerel fillets

Heat the oil in a large frying pan and sweat the onion and garlic for 5 minutes or until they have softened. Add the cabbage and some seasoning and stir-fry for 2-3 minutes. Remove the skin from the mackerel and flake the flesh into the pan for the last minute of cooking.

Tip: you can use other smoked fish for this recipe but you may need to add extra pepper and perhaps a scattering of chilli to enhance the flavours.

- **CALORIES 280**
- PROTEIN 13G
- FAT 22G
- FIBRE 4G
- CARBS 9G

Chicken biriani with cauli rice

Cauliflower rice works brilliantly with chicken biriani and dramatically reduces the amount of starchy carbohydrates involved.

Serves 4

1 large cauliflower, grated
3 tbsp coconut oil (or 50g butter)
25g flaked almonds
2 large onions, 1 sliced finely into rings, 1 diced
2 garlic cloves, finely chopped
2cm root ginger, grated
Seeds from 3 cardamom pods
1 cinnamon stick, broken in half
1 tsp turmeric
2-3 tbsp medium curry paste
4 medium skinless chicken breasts, cut into 2cm chunks
85g raisins
50-100ml chicken stock
Generous handful of coriander, chopped

Preheat the oven to 180°C. Drizzle 1 tbsp oil over the grated cauliflower, spread it out on a baking sheet and bake it in the oven for 10 minutes, shaking the tray and turning the cauliflower a few times during cooking.

Meanwhile, toast the almond flakes in a dry non-stick frying pan for a few minutes until they start to turn golden brown, then set them aside. Using the same pan, gently fry the onion rings in 1 tbsp oil until they are golden brown, then set them aside too.

In another large non-stick saucepan, heat 1 tbsp oil and fry the diced onions, garlic, ginger and spices for 5-10 minutes or until the onions are golden brown. Remove this mixture to a bowl and use the same pan to fry the chicken with the curry paste in the remaining oil. Once the chicken is cooked – this should take 5-10 minutes – stir in the cauliflower rice along with the raisins, stock and spicy onion mix. Cover the pan and simmer gently for 4-5 minutes, then stir through half the coriander. Top the biriani with the fried onion rings, the rest of the coriander and the toasted almonds. Serve with raitha (see page 72) and some steamed greens.

- **CALORIES** 390
- PROTEIN 32G
- FAT 17G
- FIBRE 4G
- CARBS 29G

Courgetti puttanesca, *see page 110*

Guilt-free spaghetti

Despite being part of the Mediterranean diet, pasta is a high-GI, starchy food that is broken down rapidly into sugars. And unfortunately brown pasta is not much better.

For those of us trying to find alternatives to pasta, a spiraliser, which looks a bit like a giant serrated pencil sharpener and shreds chunks of veg into wonderful strands of 'vegetti', has become one of the must-have pieces of kitchen equipment. We have a fairly low-tech kitchen – most of the gadgets we do have lurk somewhere towards the back of the kitchen drawers. But the spiraliser is still right up there at the front. It works best on firm vegetables like carrots, courgettes, butternut squash, celeriac (and if this all sounds too much like hard work, the good news is that you can now buy pre-prepared spiralised veg from most supermarkets).

Other spaghetti alternatives:
Konjac-based low-carb noodles (see page 198)
Finely sliced cabbage, steamed or boiled
Runner beans, shredded lengthwise (available in some supermarkets, frozen is fine)

Courgetti 6 ways

1. With pesto, goat's cheese and peas

Serves 2

200g frozen peas
1 tbsp pine nuts
3 tbsp pesto sauce (either home-made, see pg 177; or from a jar)
2 large courgettes (about 200g each), spiralised
50g goat's cheese

Boil the peas for 4-5 minutes, then drain them and set them aside. In a dry non-stick frying pan, toast the pine nuts until they turn golden at the edges (1-2 minutes) and set them aside. Steam, microwave or boil the courgetti for about 2 minutes or until it is al dente. In a bowl, mix together the courgetti, peas and pesto, then crumble in the goat's cheese and stir gently. Sprinkle the toasted pine nuts on top and serve.

- **CALORIES** 430
- PROTEIN 23G
- FAT 31G
- FIBRE 6G
- CARBS 13G

2. With bacon and beans

Serves 2

100g diced bacon, lardons or pancetta
1 tbsp olive oil
1 garlic clove, crushed
150g tinned broad beans or other beans, such as cannellini or haricot, drained and rinsed
2 heaped tbsp crème fraîche
2 large courgettes (about 200g each), spiralised
Small handful of parsley, chopped
1 tbsp Parmesan, grated

Gently fry the bacon in the olive oil in a medium-sized frying pan until it is slightly browned, then turn down the heat and add the garlic and the broad beans. Sauté for a few more minutes then remove the pan from the heat and allow the mixture to cool for a few minutes before stirring in the crème fraîche.

Steam, microwave or boil the courgetti for 2-3 minutes or until it is al dente. Mix all the cooked ingredients in a bowl, then add the parsley and scatter over the Parmesan.

Tip: we use tinned beans but you can use frozen or fresh (which will need cooking first).

- **CALORIES** 280
- PROTEIN 17G
- FAT 20G
- FIBRE 5G
- CARBS 8G

---

3. With seafood

This tastes of holidays beside the sea – it's been my favourite pasta dish since I was a teenager. And now it's got even better.

Serves 2

1 tbsp olive oil
2 garlic cloves, finely sliced
Pinch of dried chilli flakes
350g frozen mixed seafood
25g samphire (or green beans), lightly chopped
Zest of half a lemon
2 large courgettes (about 200g each), spiralised
1 tbsp pine nuts, toasted
Handful of basil leaves, torn (or 1 tsp dried basil)

Heat the oil in a medium-sized frying pan and sweat the garlic with the chilli for a few minutes until it has softened. Add the seafood and cook gently for a further 3 minutes. Then add the samphire or beans and cook for 2-3 more minutes. Give the pan a good shake to distribute the ingredients evenly and then sprinkle on the lemon zest.

Steam, microwave or boil the courgetti for 2-3 minutes or until it is al dente. Season and serve it with the seafood piled on top, and the pine nuts and basil sprinkled over.

- **CALORIES** 240
- PROTEIN 30G
- FAT 10G
- FIBRE 1G
- CARBS 9G

4. With tomato meatballs

A classic dish, now with a healthy spiralised twist.

Serves 2

200g minced beef (or any other mince)
50g Parmesan, grated
1 onion, finely diced
1 egg, beaten
½ tbsp Worcestershire sauce (or other flavouring depending on the meat)
Small handful of parsley, finely chopped
2 tbsp olive oil
Pinch of dried oregano or thyme
1 garlic clove, crushed
½ tsp chilli flakes
400g tin tomatoes
2 large courgettes (about 200g each), spiralised

In a bowl, mix the mince, half the Parmesan, half the onion, egg, Worcestershire sauce and parsley and season well. With your hands, work at the mixture for a few minutes, squidging the ingredients together and mopping up the egg to bind it. Divide it into plum-sized balls and put them in the fridge to firm up for 20 minutes before frying.

To make the tomato sauce, in a medium-sized saucepan, sweat the rest of the onion in 1 tbsp olive oil for 5 minutes, then stir in the herbs, garlic and chilli. After 2 more minutes, add the tomatoes. Simmer, uncovered, for about 20 minutes until the sauce has thickened and reduced.

Fry the meatballs in a separate frying pan in 1 tbsp olive oil for about 5 minutes, then add them to the simmering tomato sauce, to finish cooking.

Steam, microwave or boil the courgetti for 2-3 minutes or until it is al dente. Serve it with the tomato meatballs on top, scattered with the remaining Parmesan.

- **CALORIES** 400
- PROTEIN 40G
- FAT 21G
- FIBRE 3G
- CARBS 15G

5. Carbonara

Serves 2

30g Parmesan, grated
2 large egg yolks
4 tbsp double cream
50g turkey bacon, diced
1 tbsp olive oil
1 garlic clove, crushed
2 large courgettes (about 200g each), spiralised

Grate most of the cheese into a bowl, add the egg yolks and cream, season with black pepper and whisk everything together.

In a medium-sized saucepan, fry the bacon in the olive oil for 4-5 minutes, then add the garlic and courgetti and cook for a further few minutes. Stir in the sauce, ensuring that everything is well coated, and serve with the remainder of the Parmesan sprinkled on top.

- **CALORIES** 500
- PROTEIN 16G
- FAT 47G
- FIBRE 1G
- CARBS 4G

---

6. Puttanesca

Full of healthy Mediterranean ingredients, including anchovies, which bring a delicate salty taste. Excellent for reluctant fish eaters.

Serves 2

4 anchovies from a jar or tin, drained and chopped
1 garlic clove, crushed
2 tbsp olive oil
¼-½ tsp chilli flakes or fresh chilli, deseeded and finely diced
½ 400g tin chopped tomatoes
2 tbsp capers, rinsed
50g pitted black olives, sliced
1 tsp dried oregano
2 large courgettes (about 200g each), spiralised

Over a gentle heat, fry the anchovies, garlic and chilli in the oil for 2-3 minutes. Press the anchovies against the pan with a wooden spoon to form a paste. Then add the tomatoes, capers and olives and cook gently for 20-30 minutes without a lid. About 5 minutes before the sauce is ready, steam, microwave or boil the courgetti for 2-3 minutes, so that it is still slightly al dente. Serve the sauce on top of the courgetti along with a light salad.

- **CALORIES** 170
- PROTEIN 5G
- FAT 15G
- FIBRE 2G
- CARBS 5G

Prawn and tuna fried rice

This delicious seafood fried rice can be made almost entirely from items that you are likely to have in store.

Serves 2

½ tbsp coconut or rapeseed oil
1 onion, chopped
½ tsp chilli flakes or fresh chilli, deseeded and finely diced (to taste)
1 garlic clove, chopped
1cm root ginger, chopped
1 red pepper, deseeded and chopped
200g cauliflower rice (see page 98)
100g prawns (raw or frozen, defrosted)
100g tinned tuna
1 tbsp Thai fish sauce
200g Chinese vegetables or cabbage, diced
2 eggs, beaten
Handful of coriander, torn

Heat the oil in a wok and fry the onion, chilli, garlic and ginger for 1-2 minutes before adding the red pepper and, after 4-5 minutes, the cauliflower rice. After a couple more minutes, stir in the prawns, tuna, fish sauce and the Chinese vegetables or cabbage. (If using fresh prawns, cook them until they are pink before adding the other ingredients.) Continue to fry gently for another few minutes. Finally, clear a hollow in the centre of the wok in which to scramble the eggs. Stir them though, season and garnish the dish with the coriander.

- **CALORIES** 290
- PROTEIN 34G
- FAT 12G
- FIBRE 5G
- CARBS 13G

High-protein salads

These salads are all potentially meals in themselves. You don't need to stick to the exact ingredients – go with what you have to hand or what is in season.

Watercress, orange and sardine salad

A wonderful combination of flavours and textures – even better with fresh sardines.

Serves 2

2 oranges (including the zest of one)
1 tbsp olive oil
Juice of half a lemon
100g watercress
½ red onion, thinly sliced
Handful of tarragon or coriander leaves, torn
120g tin sardines in oil, drained (or fresh sardines if available, see tip)
1 tbsp pumpkin seeds

In a bowl, make a dressing by whisking together the orange zest, oil and lemon juice with some salt and pepper. Peel both oranges, removing as much pith as possible, and cut them into slices. Arrange the watercress, onion and tarragon leaves in a bowl, add the slices of orange and then the sardines. Drizzle over the dressing and sprinkle with pumpkin seeds.

Tip: if you have a good fishmonger, it is well worth using fresh sardines (allow 2 per person). Buy them scaled and gutted, with heads and gills removed. Rub them with olive oil, generous amounts of salt and ground pepper, and cook them on a griddle for about 5 minutes, turning once. They are cooked if the flesh in the thickest part of the fish pulls away easily.

- CALORIES 320
- PROTEIN 19G
- FAT 19G
- FIBRE 4G
- CARBS 19G

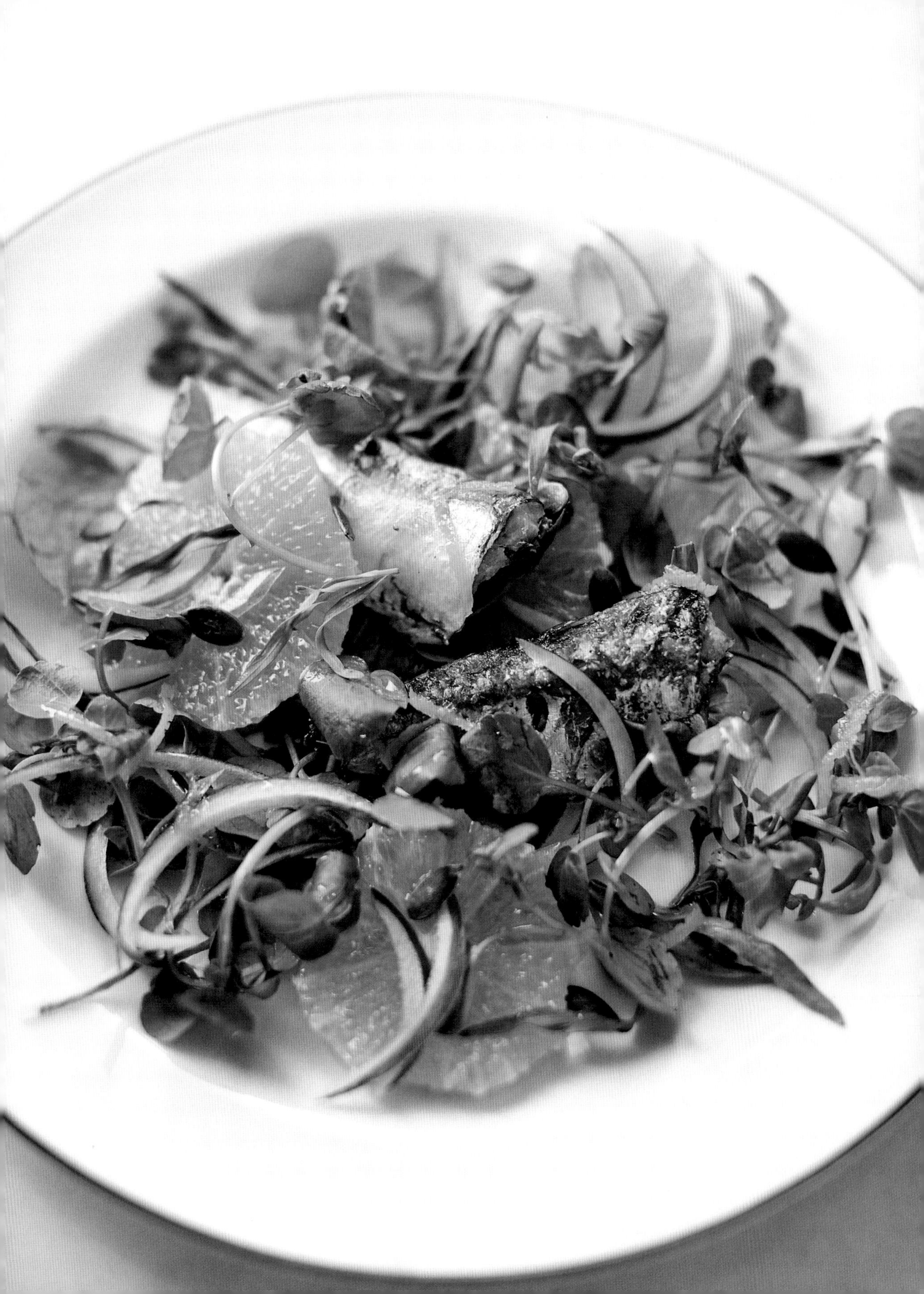

Chicory 2 ways

Chicory is a wonderful vegetable, providing the nutritional benefits that often come with bitter foods. Sadly, it is too sharp a flavour for modern tastes. Chicory also has high levels of inulin, a form of fibre which encourages the growth of healthy bacteria in your gut. All good to keep the sugars down.

1. With anchovy mayo

The slight bitterness of the chicory is counteracted by the creamy mayonnaise here. A delicious and interesting combination.

Serves 2

1 tbsp full-fat mayonnaise
1 tbsp extra-virgin olive oil
1 tbsp lime juice
1 level tbsp rosemary leaves, very finely chopped
3 anchovy fillets from a jar or tin, finely diced
2 heads of chicory
Large handful of rocket or baby lettuce leaves
½ red pepper, deseeded and diced (optional)

Mix the mayonnaise, oil and lime well, then add the rosemary and anchovies and blitz with a hand blender or mix together energetically with a spoon to infuse the flavours. Discard the outer leaves of the chicory and separate the rest from the stalk. Arrange the leaves on a serving plate with the rocket or lettuce and the red pepper, if using. Drizzle over the anchovy dressing and season generously with freshly ground black pepper.

- CALORIES 170
- PROTEIN 3G
- FAT 16G
- FIBRE 2G
- CARBS 6G

2. Chicory, pear, hazelnut and goat's cheese salad

Serves 2

2 tbsp olive oil
1 tbsp cider vinegar
2 heads of chicory
1 pear, cored and sliced
60g goat's cheese, diced
Handful of rocket leaves
2 tbsp hazelnuts, toasted

In a bowl, make a dressing by whisking together the oil and vinegar with some salt and pepper. Discard the outer leaves of the chicory and separate the rest from the stalk. Arrange the leaves on 2 plates, with the pear slices and cheese on top. Drizzle over the dressing and scatter the rocket leaves and nuts on top.

- CALORIES 310
- PROTEIN 9G
- FAT 26G
- FIBRE 4G
- CARBS 12G

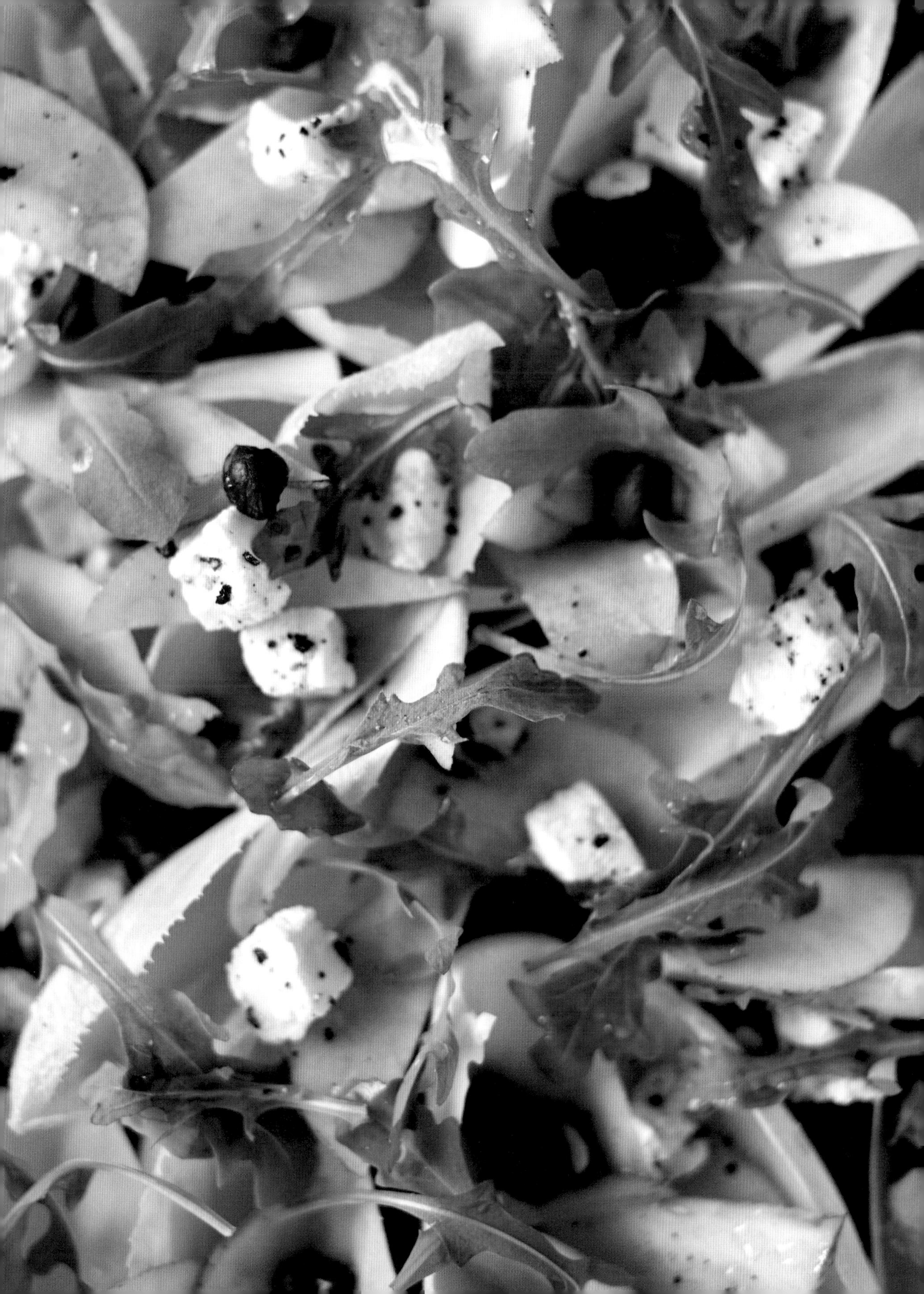

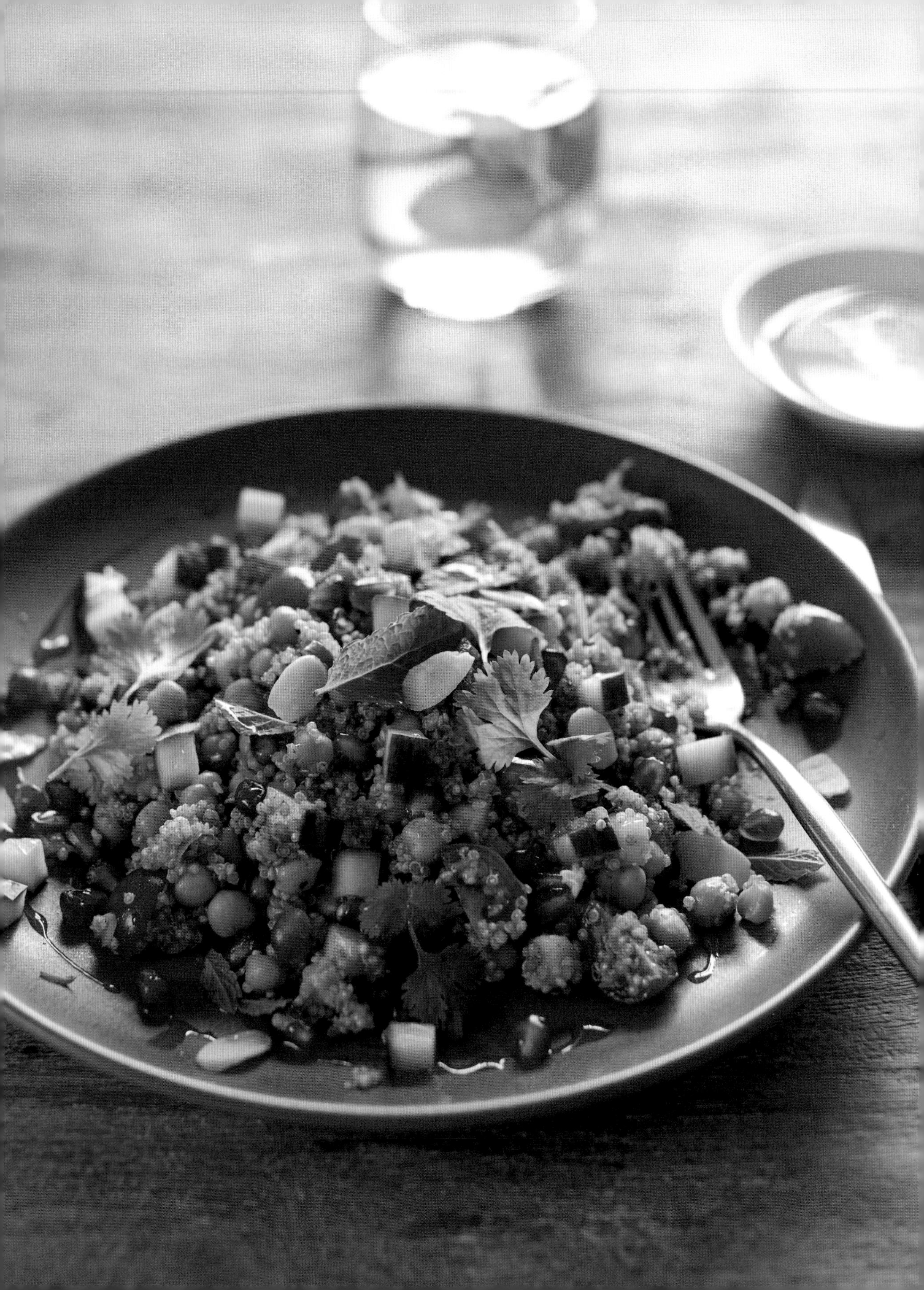

Moroccan spiced chickpea salad

We use quinoa here instead of couscous as it is higher in protein and fibre and significantly lower in starchy carbohydrates.

Serves 4

200g quinoa (mixture of dark and pale if available)
350ml vegetable stock
400g tin chickpeas, drained and rinsed
1 tbsp olive oil
Juice of 1 lemon
1 tsp ras el hanout (or harissa paste or paprika)
8 cherry tomatoes, halved
¼ cucumber, deseeded and diced
4 spring onions, finely chopped
100g pomegranate seeds (or raisins)
Handful of mint or coriander leaves, torn
2 tbsp flaked almonds, toasted

Place the quinoa in a saucepan with the stock, bring it to the boil, then reduce the heat and simmer for 10-15 minutes or until all the stock has been absorbed. Remove it from the heat, cover it and leave it to stand for 5 more minutes.

Put the chickpeas into a wide bowl and add the oil, lemon and spice. Mix well to coat the chickpeas. Add the quinoa and all the other ingredients to the chickpeas and gently toss them together. Season with salt and freshly ground black pepper.

Tip: deseed the cucumber by cutting it in half lengthwise and scooping out the watery seeds with a teaspoon.

- **CALORIES** 400
- PROTEIN 15G
- FAT 14G
- FIBRE 8G
- CARBS 60G

Lentil, carrot and avocado salad

A perfect combination of Mediterranean goodness.

Serves 2

1 tbsp olive oil
300g carrots, cut into batons
1 tsp cumin seeds
100g tinned Puy lentils, rinsed and drained
2 handfuls of lamb's lettuce leaves
1 avocado, sliced
2 tsp sesame seeds
1 tbsp raisins
Juice of half a lemon (or 1 tbsp cider vinegar)

Preheat the oven to 200°C. Toss the carrots in the oil and cumin seeds in a baking tray and roast them for 20 minutes. Leave them to cool for a few minutes. Place the lettuce in a bowl with the lentils and avocado. Add the carrots and sprinkle over the sesame seeds and raisins, followed by a generous squeeze of lemon and some salt and black pepper.

Tip: to convert this salad into a more substantial meal, you could add a handful of nuts and/or a handful of feta, and adjust the calories accordingly.

- **CALORIES** 330
- PROTEIN 8G
- FAT 20G
- FIBRE 8G
- CARBS 31G

Prawn, pea and spring onion salad

A lovely light summery salad.

Serves 2

100g frozen peas
Juice and zest of half a lemon
100ml crème fraîche
Handful of chives, snipped
2 gem lettuces, chopped
200g cooked prawns
3 spring onions, finely sliced

Cook the peas in a pan of boiling water for 5 minutes. Drain them, run them under cold water and set them aside. Whisk the lemon zest and juice with the crème fraîche, season with salt and pepper and stir in the chives. Place the lettuce in a bowl, add the prawns, peas and spring onions and toss everything in the chive dressing.

- **CALORIES** 300
- PROTEIN 20G
- FAT 21G
- FIBRE 3G
- CARBS 8G

Roasted beetroot and fig salad

The tangy beetroot is a perfect foil for the sweet figs and salty feta.

Serves 2

2 large beetroots (about 300g), chopped into chunks or wedges
1 red onion, quartered
2 tbsp olive oil
2 tbsp balsamic vinegar
2 ripe figs, quartered
30g walnuts or hazelnuts, roughly chopped
50g feta
Generous handful of basil leaves, torn

Preheat the oven to 200°C. Spread the beetroot and onion on a baking tray, drizzle over the olive oil and balsamic vinegar and season with salt and pepper. Cover the tray with foil and place it in the oven. After 20 minutes stir in the figs and walnuts and return it to the oven, uncovered, for another 20 minutes. When the mixture has cooled, crumble the feta over it and stir in the basil.

Tip: wear rubber gloves when you peel and cut the beetroot as it will stain your fingers.

- **CALORIES** 210
- PROTEIN 4G
- FAT 14G
- FIBRE 3G
- CARBS 18G

Crunchy red coleslaw with minute steak

Serves 2

2 small steaks such as skirt or sirloin, beaten thinner
½ small red cabbage, outer leaves removed
1 carrot
1 red apple
4 spring onions, finely sliced
1 tbsp olive oil
1 tbsp cider vinegar
2 tbsp mayonnaise

Season the steaks with salt and pepper (or a sprinkle of steak seasoning). Finely shred the cabbage and place it in a bowl. Grate the carrot and apple into the bowl and add the spring onions. Make a dressing by whisking together the oil, vinegar and mayonnaise and stir it through the cabbage mixture. Heat a griddle pan and cook the steaks to your liking. Slice them diagonally and serve them with the coleslaw.

- **CALORIES** 430
- PROTEIN 23G
- FAT 31G
- FIBRE 5G
- CARBS 14G

Main Meals

These are more substantial recipes suited to occasions when you have extra time for cooking, perhaps at the weekend or when family and friends are around.

As you know, we Blood Sugar dieters are trying to avoid using starchy carbohydrates wherever possible. Fortunately, there are lots of tasty and filling alternatives so you should be able to keep everyone happy. Cauliflower mash is a brilliant substitute for mashed potato, astonishingly low in starchy carbohydrate. Beans and lentils are great for thickening casseroles and stews. And there are all sorts of healthy toppings you can use on bakes, pies and gratins – those ideal one-pot meals, ready the moment you pull them out of the oven.

Michael's easy roast chicken, see page 155

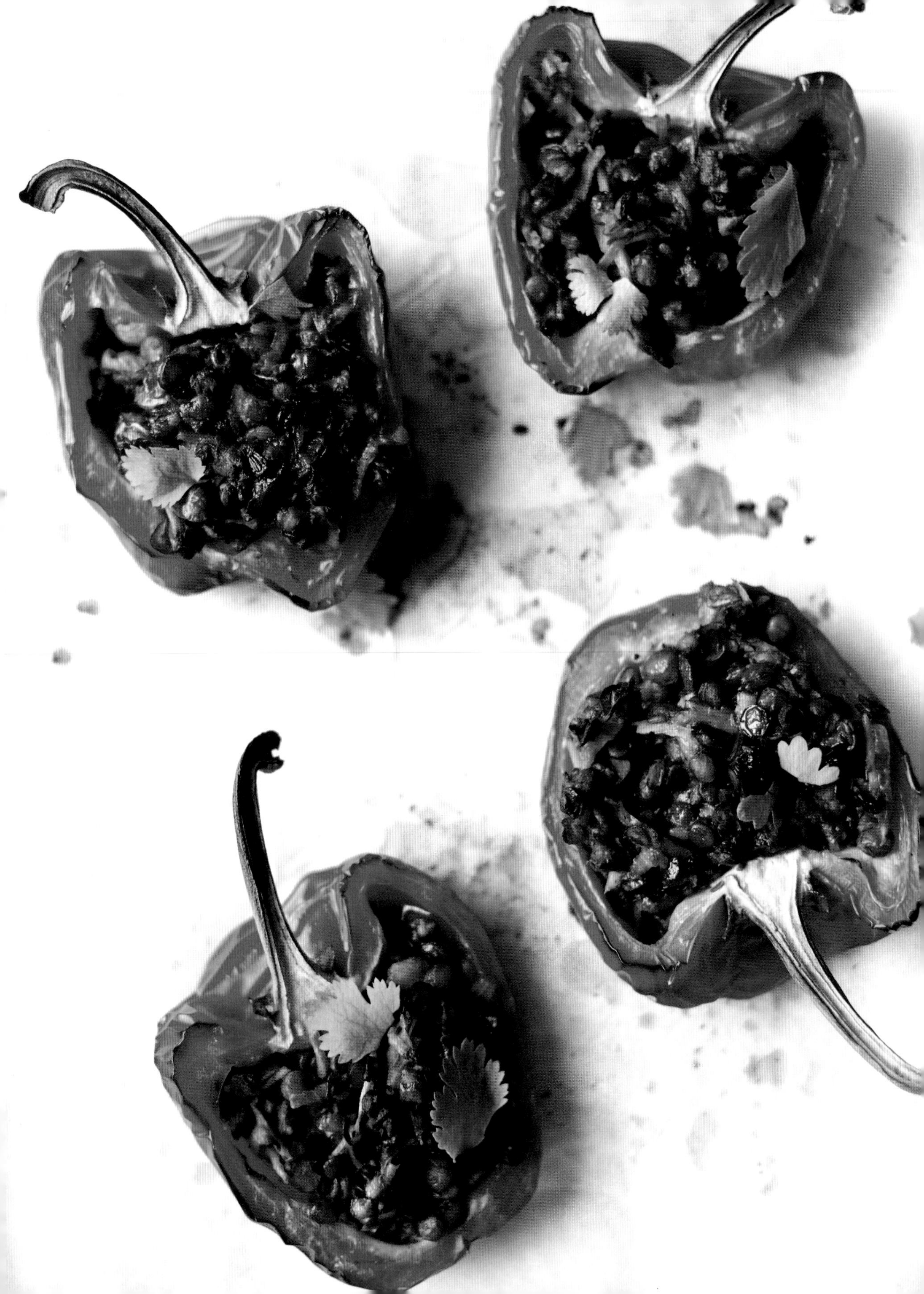

Spicy stuffed red pepper

This recipe was contributed by our great friends Drs Rajsingh and Rai who specialise in healthy Indian food. The dahl stuffing has an exotic nutty flavour, spicy but not hot, and works well eaten hot or cold.

Serves 2

2 medium onions, chopped
2 tbsp vegetable or olive oil
250g pack microwaveable Puy lentils (or 400g tin green lentils, drained and rinsed)
3-4 garlic cloves, diced (or 2 tsp garlic paste)
4cm root ginger, diced (or 1 tsp ginger paste)
2 bay leaves
2 cinnamon sticks
2 cardamom pods
1 tsp ground cumin or seeds
1 chilli, diced, or 1 tsp chilli flakes (to taste)
Handful of coriander, chopped
Juice of 1 lime
2 large red peppers, halved lengthwise and deseeded

Preheat the oven to 180°C. Heat 1 tbsp oil in a saucepan and sweat the onions for about 5 minutes, or until they start to turn golden brown. Meanwhile, put the lentils, garlic, ginger, bay leaves, cinnamon sticks, cardamoms, cumin and chilli in a medium-sized bowl and mix them together. Season with salt and pepper.

When the onions are ready, add the lentil mixture and simmer on a low heat for 8-10 minutes, before stirring in the coriander and lime juice. Then fill the pepper halves with the mixture and place them on a greased baking tray with the open side facing up. Drizzle the remaining olive oil over them, cover them with foil and bake them for 10 minutes. Remove the foil and bake them for a further 10 minutes.

Tips: with the flat of a knife gently crush the cardamom pod to release the flavour. If you prefer you can prepare the green lentils from scratch, using 80g dried lentils (see page 196).

- **CALORIES** 240
- PROTEIN 6G
- FAT 13G
- FIBRE 8G
- CARBS 28G

Easy Bolognese

This is a great foolproof Bolognese, and makes a fairly large batch from which you can save or freeze portions to create all sorts of other dishes – see no-pasta beef 'lasagne' and chilli con carne (opposite).

Serves 6

1 tbsp olive oil
1 onion, finely diced
450g minced beef (or Quorn mince for vegetarians)
1 garlic clove, diced
2 heaped tsp dried oregano
2 medium carrots, grated
2 x 400g tins chopped tomatoes
1 beef stock cube
2 tbsp tomato purée
½ tbsp Worcestershire sauce
½ tsp chilli flakes (to taste)
3 bay leaves

In a medium-sized casserole, sweat the onion in the olive oil until it is golden brown – about 5 minutes. Add the mince, garlic and oregano and cook until the meat is lightly browned.

Stir in the rest of the ingredients, cover the pan and simmer gently for about an hour, stirring occasionally and adding a little water if it's looking dry. Serve with steamed or boiled finely sliced cabbage, courgetti (see page 107), or konjack noodles (see page 198).

- **CALORIES** 170
- PROTEIN 17G
- FAT 9G
- FIBRE 1G
- CARBS 5G

Chilli con carne

Use the Bolognese (left) as a base and simply add these extra ingredients, adjusting the proportions according to how much Bolognese you are converting. So if you have half left, use half the quantities below.

Serves 6

1 tbsp cocoa powder (not drinking chocolate which is full of sugar!)
1 tsp ground cumin
1 tsp ground coriander
1 red pepper, deseeded and finely diced
200g mushrooms, sliced
400g tin kidney beans or black beans, drained and rinsed
1 tsp chilli, diced, or chilli flakes (to taste)
Soured cream, to serve

Stir all the ingredients except the soured cream into the Bolognese base, cover the pan and simmer for 15-20 minutes, adding water if it starts to dry out. Serve with a dollop of soured cream on top, and steamed finely sliced cabbage or cauliflower rice (see page 98).

- **CALORIES** 260
- PROTEIN 23G
- FAT 1G
- FIBRE 7G
- CARBS 19G

No-pasta beef 'lasagne'

A delicious low-carb lasagne, in which the stodgy sheets of pasta are replaced with red cabbage leaves. Our daughter was horrified at the thought of cabbage in a lasagne, but it works surprisingly well. Try it and see.

Serves 6

4 x portions of Bolognese sauce (see recipe opposite)
100g outer leaves of red cabbage (or white)

For the white sauce:
250g ricotta
250g crème fraîche
50g Parmesan, grated
100g spinach
½ tsp nutmeg
100g Cheddar, grated

Preheat the oven to 150°C. In a pan, heat the Bolognese sauce and transfer it to a large baking dish. Cut each cabbage leaf in half and remove the tough central stalk, taking care not to tear the rest of the leaf. Lay a single layer of cabbage leaves over the Bolognese sauce, overlapping them slightly to keep the Bolognese separate from the creamy sauce to be added next.

Mix the ricotta, crème fraîche and Parmesan in a bowl and stir in the spinach. Add the nutmeg and some ground black pepper, then dollop the mixture over the layer of red cabbage. Sprinkle the grated Cheddar on top and bake it in the oven for 30-40 minutes.

- **CALORIES** 500
- PROTEIN 29G
- FAT 38G
- FIBRE 2G
- CARBS 10G

Michael's Thai fish cakes

Michael has whipped these fish cakes together with great speed and in large quantities for several parties, but they are also perfect for a light meal. They have a great texture and an exotic flavour and, because we use chia seeds rather than flour or breadcrumbs to bind the mixture, they are less starchy and more nutritious.

Serves 2

200g white fish fillets, skinned and cut into chunks
1 small egg
2 tsp Thai red curry paste (to taste)
½ tbsp Thai fish sauce
¼ tsp lime zest, finely shredded
1 spring onion, finely diced (set aside 1 tsp for the dipping sauce)
1 tbsp coriander, finely chopped
2 tsp chia seeds
1 tbsp coconut or rapeseed oil

For the sweet and sour dipping sauce:
2-3 tsp sweet chilli sauce (see page 175)
1 tsp Thai fish sauce
1 tsp cider vinegar
2 tsp water
20g cucumber, deseeded and very finely diced

Put the sauce ingredients in a small saucepan and bring them to the boil, then simmer for about 1 minute. Pour the sauce into 2 small bowls.

Drain any fluid from the fish and blend it with the rest of the ingredients either in a food processor or with a hand blender until you have a slightly rough texture. Place the mixture in the fridge for 10 minutes to firm it up a little, then divide it into 4. Flatten each piece into a patty.

Heat the oil in a frying pan and fry the patties on a medium heat for 2-3 minutes on each side or until they are golden brown. Serve with the dipping sauce and cabbage stir-fried Chinese style (see page 169) or Swiss chard stir-fried with garlic (see pg 168).

- **CALORIES** 130
- PROTEIN 21G
- FAT 3G
- FIBRE 0G
- CARBS 4G

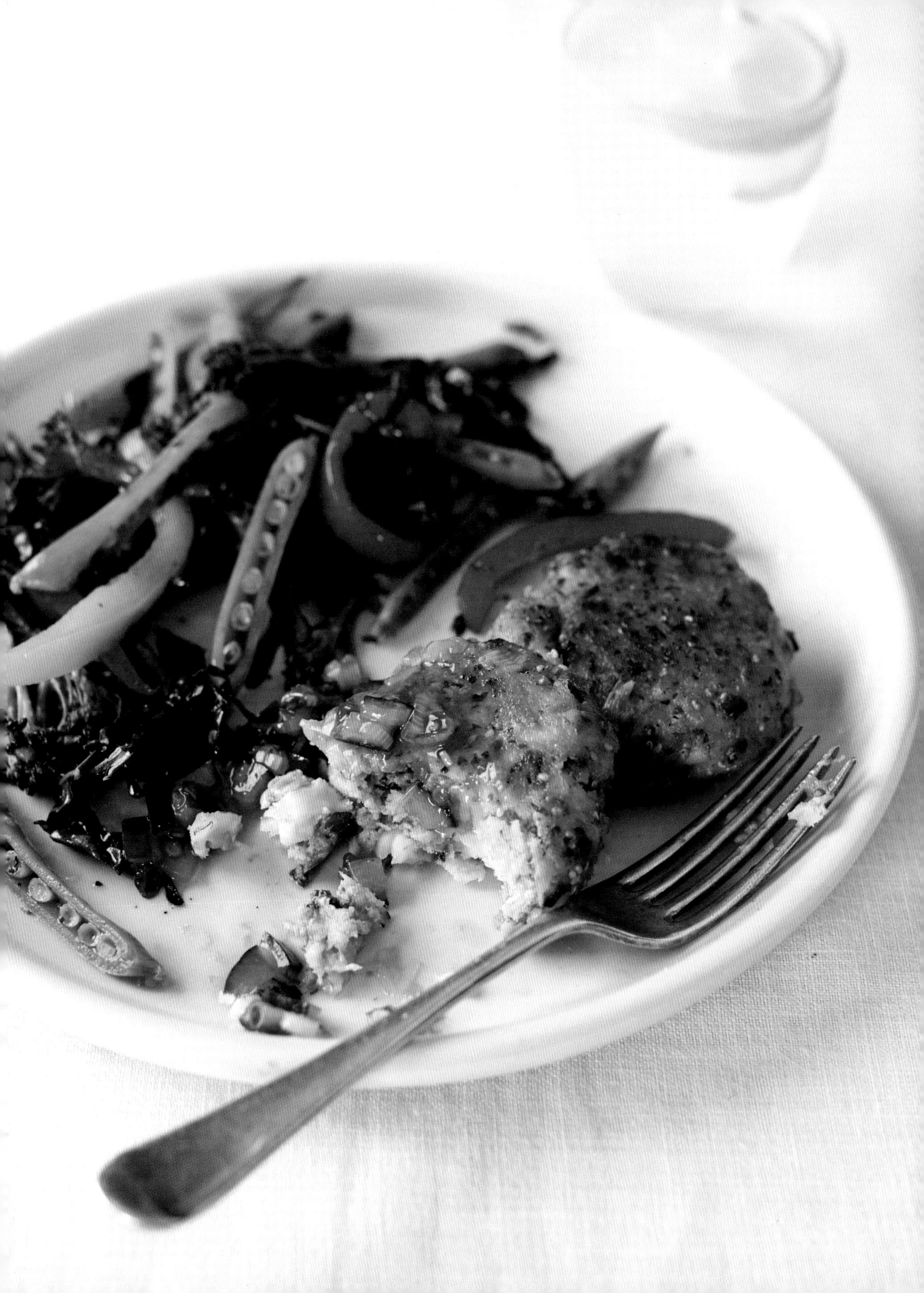

Pork steaks in mustard sauce

These are wonderfully quick and easy to prepare. The creamy mustard sauce soaks up the juices and complements the pork deliciously.

Serves 2

½ tbsp olive oil
2 boneless pork steaks
2 generous tsp mustard (wholegrain or Dijon)
2 level tbsp crème fraîche
Small handful of parsley, chopped

Fry the pork steaks in the oil in a small frying pan for 15-20 minutes, or until the juices do not run pink. Take the pan off the heat, allow the meat to cool for a few minutes and then add the mustard and crème fraîche, stirring them into the juices. Season and scatter the parsley over.

Serve with 2 tbsp cooked grains such as quinoa or bulgar wheat to soak up the juices (see page 99) and green veg.

- **CALORIES** 290
- PROTEIN 25G
- FAT 20G
- FIBRE 0G
- CARBS 2G

Bulgar wheat risotto with chicken and artichokes

Bulgar wheat is a wholegrain cereal which has been parboiled, allowing it to be cooked more quickly, and retain a fairly high fibre content. This 'risotto' is also an excellent way to use up leftover chicken.

Serves 2

1 onion, finely chopped
1 tbsp olive oil
1 large garlic clove, diced or squeezed
60g bulgar wheat
½-1 red chilli, diced, or ½ tsp chilli flakes (to taste)
1 bay leaf
1 red pepper, deseeded and sliced
300ml chicken or vegetable stock
140g cooked leftover chicken, chopped (about 1 medium chicken breast)
2 heaped tbsp artichokes (from a jar or tin), quartered
Large handful of coriander or parsley, roughly chopped

Sweat the onions and garlic in the olive oil in a saucepan. Add the bulgar wheat, chilli, bay leaf and red pepper and cover with around 2cm stock. Put the lid on and let it simmer for 20-25 minutes or until most of the fluid has been absorbed and the bulgar wheat is al dente. Check every now and again and add extra stock if it is looking dry.

Then stir the chicken into the pan, along with the artichokes, for the last 5-10 minutes of cooking. Season and stir in half the coriander, reserving the rest to garnish.

Tip: this also works really well if you swap the chicken for 60g fried sliced halloumi.

- **CALORIES** 330
- PROTEIN 22G
- FAT 12G
- FIBRE 2G
- CARBS 35G

Garlic and rosemary fried lamb

Full of Mediterranean flavours and so easy to prepare, this lamb is delicious served with quinoa. Quinoa is great for occasional use on the Blood Sugar Diet as it has far more protein and fibre than rice and therefore a lower impact on blood sugar (see page 99).

Serves 2

2 sprigs of rosemary, leaves only
1 garlic clove
Squeeze of lemon juice
1 tbsp olive oil
2 lamb chops, or medium-sized lamb steaks
60g quinoa (the darker variety if available)
200ml chicken or vegetable stock
¼ cucumber, cut in half lengthwise and deseeded

Use a pestle and mortar (or a spoon in a bowl) to crush together the garlic and rosemary leaves with a drizzle of olive oil and the lemon juice. Place the lamb chops in a dish, pour over the marinade and spread it over the surface of the meat.

Put the quinoa in a small saucepan, cover it with 1-2cm stock and bring it to the boil. Then immediately put the lid on and turn down the heat. Simmer for 10 minutes or until the liquid has been absorbed. Turn off the heat and leave it to steam with the lid on for a further 10 minutes. Dice the cucumber finely and put it aside to add to the quinoa before serving.

When the quinoa is nearly ready, season the lamb, then fry it on both sides in a drizzle of olive oil in a non-stick pan until it is slightly browned. Serve the lamb with greens or green beans and a couple of tbsp quinoa, and pour over any juices remaining in the pan.

- CALORIES 330
- PROTEIN 29G
- FAT 16G
- FIBRE 2G
- CARBS 18G

Chicken korma

One of the nation's favourites that went out of fashion in the days of low-fat diets but, hurrah, is now back on the menu.

Serves 2

2 tbsp oil
2 onions, one finely chopped, the other sliced into rings
2 garlic cloves, finely chopped
1cm root ginger, finely chopped
1 tsp garam masala
½ tsp cayenne pepper
Seeds from 4 cardamom pods
1 tsp turmeric
4 small boneless chicken thighs or 2 small chicken breasts, chopped into 1-2cm chunks
200ml coconut milk (or 200ml full-fat natural Greek yoghurt)
25g ground almonds
½ medium cauliflower, grated
Handful of coriander, roughly chopped

Heat 1 tbsp oil in an ovenproof casserole or pan and fry the finely chopped onions, garlic and ginger over a medium heat for 2-3 minutes. Add the spices and cook for 1 more minute.

Add the chicken and cook for 2-3 minutes, then pour in the coconut milk and ground almonds and simmer gently on the hob for 20 minutes. Alternatively, put the casserole in an oven preheated to 150°C for 20 minutes.

Meanwhile, heat the remaining oil in a non-stick frying pan and fry the onion rings for 5-10 minutes or until they are browned, turning them frequently. Remove the rings with a slotted spoon and place them on kitchen paper.

When the curry is nearly ready, fry the grated cauliflower gently in the oil remaining from the fried onions for 5 minutes.

Season the curry and stir in the coriander. Place the cauliflower rice on the plate, add the curry, scatter the fried onions on top and serve with 100g fine green beans.

- **CALORIES** 340
- PROTEIN 28G
- FAT 19G
- FIBRE 5G
- CARBS 17G

Thai red curry

A gently spicy, aromatic Thai curry, with a creamy sweetness thanks to the coconut milk, and quick to make if you use a shop-bought curry paste.

Serves 2

1 large chicken breast, sliced
½ onion, chopped
1 tbsp olive oil
1 large garlic clove, diced
2cm root ginger, diced
3-4 heaped tsp Thai red curry paste
1 red pepper, deseeded and sliced
½ 400ml tin coconut milk
½ tbsp Thai fish sauce
½ tsp lime zest or kaffir lime leaves (optional)
½ cauliflower, grated
Generous handful of fine beans

Heat the oil in a wok or wide-based saucepan and fry the chicken and onion. When they begin to brown, add the garlic, ginger and curry paste. Fry gently for a few minutes, then add the red pepper, coconut milk, Thai fish sauce and lime zest and cook for 15 minutes.

Meanwhile, prepare the cauliflower rice (see page 98). A few minutes before the end of cooking time, throw the green veg in the pan.

Tips: you can use prawns or tofu instead of chicken. Kaffir lime leaves can be bought fresh and kept in the freezer.

- **CALORIES** 300
- PROTEIN 4G
- FAT 25G
- FIBRE 2G
- CARBS 14G

Smoked mackerel and mushroom frittata

Serves 2

3 eggs
100g cottage cheese
25g Parmesan, grated
½ tbsp olive oil
50g mushrooms, sliced
2 spring onions, chopped
2 peppered mackerel fillets, flaked
2 large handfuls of baby-leaf spinach, chopped
½-1 tsp chilli flakes, (optional)

Preheat the grill to high. Whisk the eggs in a bowl together with the cottage cheese and the Parmesan. Season with a pinch of salt and plenty of black pepper and set to one side.

Heat the oil in an ovenproof frying pan or omelette pan. Fry the mushrooms for 3-4 minutes, then add the spring onions and mackerel and cook for another 2 minutes. Stir in the spinach and cook it until it has just wilted. Make sure the mixture is spread evenly over the pan, then pour over the eggs and a sprinkling of chilli flakes and cook gently for 4-5 minutes on the hob.

Put the pan under the grill for about 4 minutes, until the eggs have set. Serve warm with a green leafy salad.

- **CALORIES** 380
- PROTEIN 27G
- FAT 29G
- FIBRE 1G
- CARBS 2G

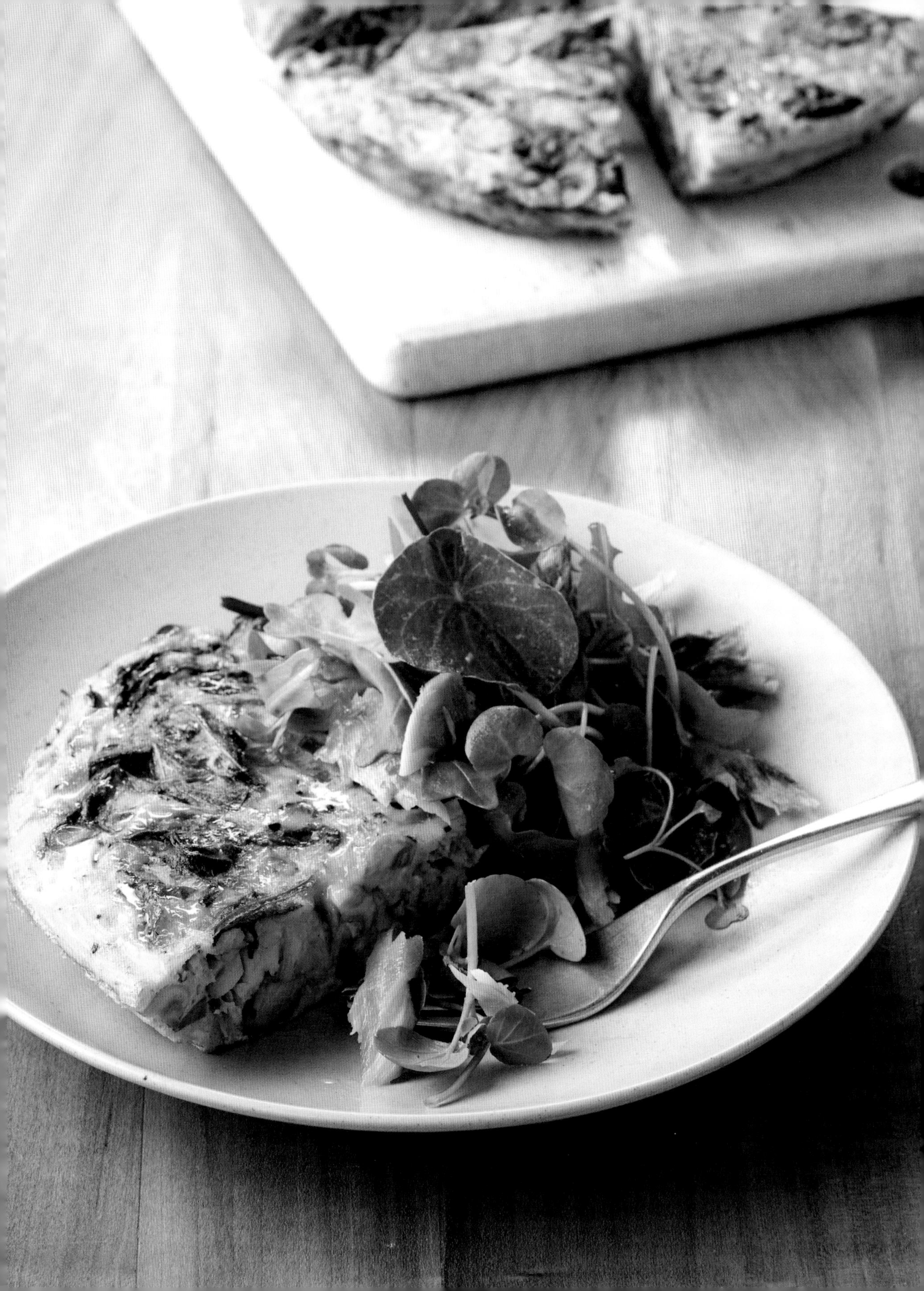

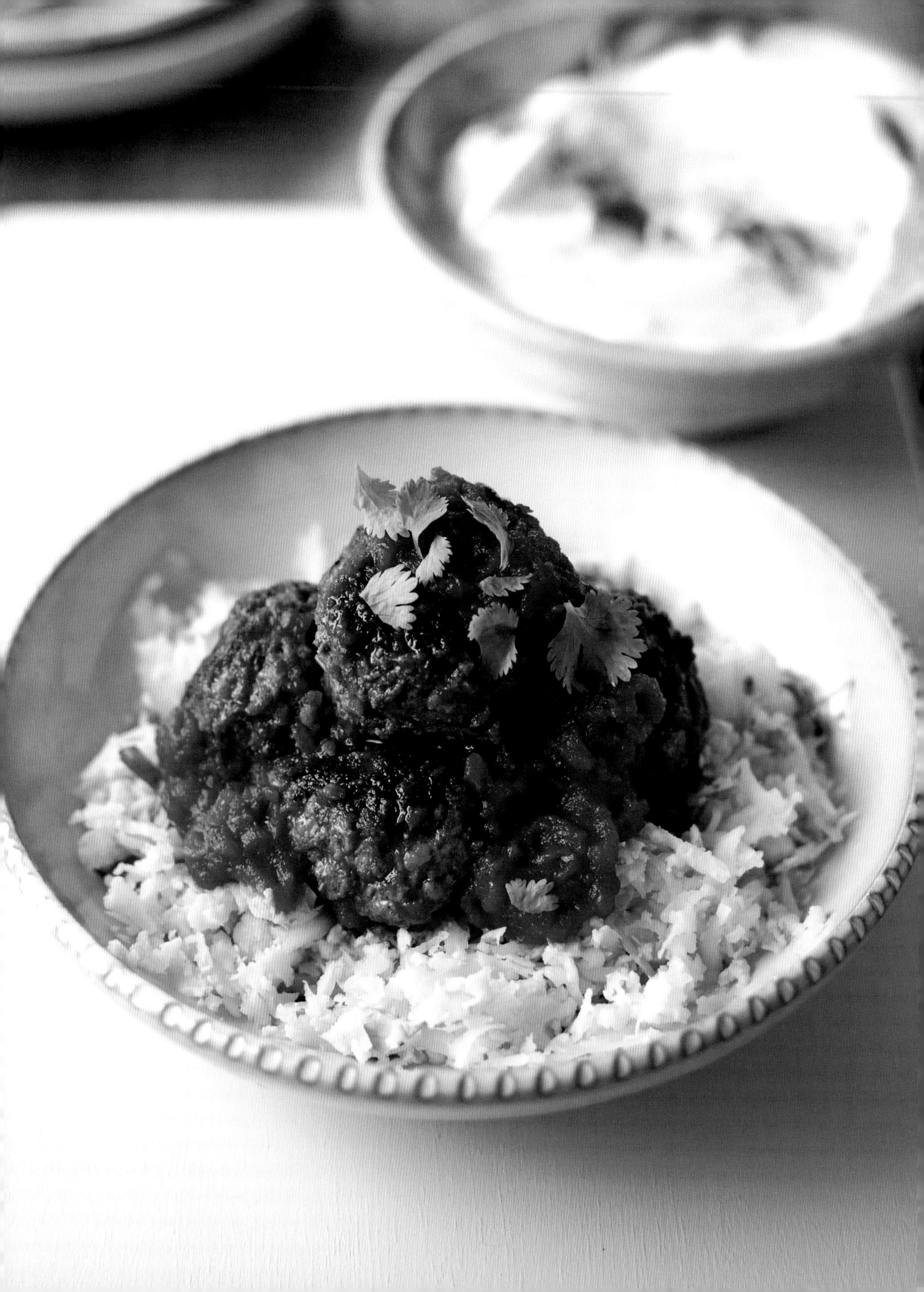

Moroccan meatballs in tomato sauce

Serves 6

1 onion, diced (half very finely for the meatballs)
400g minced lamb or beef
2 small garlic cloves, finely diced
1 egg
1 tbsp olive oil

For the tomato sauce:
1 tbsp olive oil
400g tin chopped tomatoes
½ tsp each of paprika, ground cumin, chilli flakes (or chilli paste)
Handful of coriander or parsley, chopped

Vigorously mix the mince with the finely diced onion, garlic and egg in a bowl. Season with salt and black pepper. Roll the mixture into about 16 plum-sized balls and place them in the fridge to firm up while you are preparing the sauce.

Fry the rest of the onion gently in 1 tbsp olive oil until it is golden brown, then add the tomatoes and spices. Simmer gently for 15-20 minutes.

Heat the olive oil in a large frying pan and fry the meatballs. When they are browned, add them to the sauce to cook through. Season to taste; stir in half the coriander and garnish with the rest. Serve with cauliflower rice (add 30 calories; see page 98)

Tip: alternatively, you can make these into burgers, adding the spices to the mince instead, and serve them with a salad.

- **CALORIES** 390
- PROTEIN 29G
- FAT 28G
- FIBRE 2G
- CARBS 8G

Chinese duck with green 'pancakes'

OK, I concede that it is pushing it to call lettuce a pancake... but for years we felt guilty eating duck pancakes because of the high-fat content in duck, only to realise we have been worrying about the wrong thing. It's the starchy pancakes we should avoid. The sugar in the hoisin sauce is absorbed slowly as part of the meal, so is not of much significance here.

Serves 2

2 duck legs
1 tbsp soy sauce
½ tbsp sesame oil (optional)
1 small cucumber, cut in half lengthwise and deseeded
6 spring onions
Hoisin sauce, 1 tsp per 'pancake'
Cos or little gem lettuce

Place the duck on an oven tray, score the surface with a sharp knife and rub soy sauce into the skin. Drizzle with the sesame oil if using. Leave the duck to marinate while the oven heats to 200°C. As soon as you place the duck in the oven, reduce the temperature to 160°C and roast it for an hour, turning and basting it regularly. Chop the cucumber and spring onions into matchsticks and place them on two separate plates.

The duck is ready when the flesh easily comes away from the bone. Use a spoon and fork to shred it and serve on a plate with the vegetables and lettuce 'pancakes' and a bowl of hoisin sauce.

- **CALORIES** 340
- PROTEIN 13G
- FAT 35G
- FIBRE 1G
- CARBS 5G

Low-carb pizza

Serves 1

80g celeriac, peeled and grated
2 tbsp soft cheese
1 tbsp Cheddar, grated
1 egg, beaten
1 tsp olive oil
3 tbsp tomato pizza paste, or tomato purée
2 mozzarella balls, torn
Handful of basil leaves, shredded
Handful of black olives chopped

Preheat the oven to 200°C. Place the grated celeriac in a bowl, add the cheeses and mix in the egg with some black pepper. Line a baking tray with greaseproof paper brushed with a little oil. Shape the celeriac mixture into a circle on the paper and bake it in the oven for 15 minutes.

Remove the base from the oven and allow it to cool for a minute or so before spreading the tomato paste over the surface. Then dot it with the mozzarella, basil and olives and return it to the oven for another 4-5 minutes.

Tips: use grated cauliflower instead of celeriac for the base. Add anchovies, spinach or feta or the topping of your choice. You can bake several of the bases at a time and store them in the freezer.

- **CALORIES** 490
- PROTEIN 30G
- FAT 38G
- FIBRE 4G
- CARBS 6G

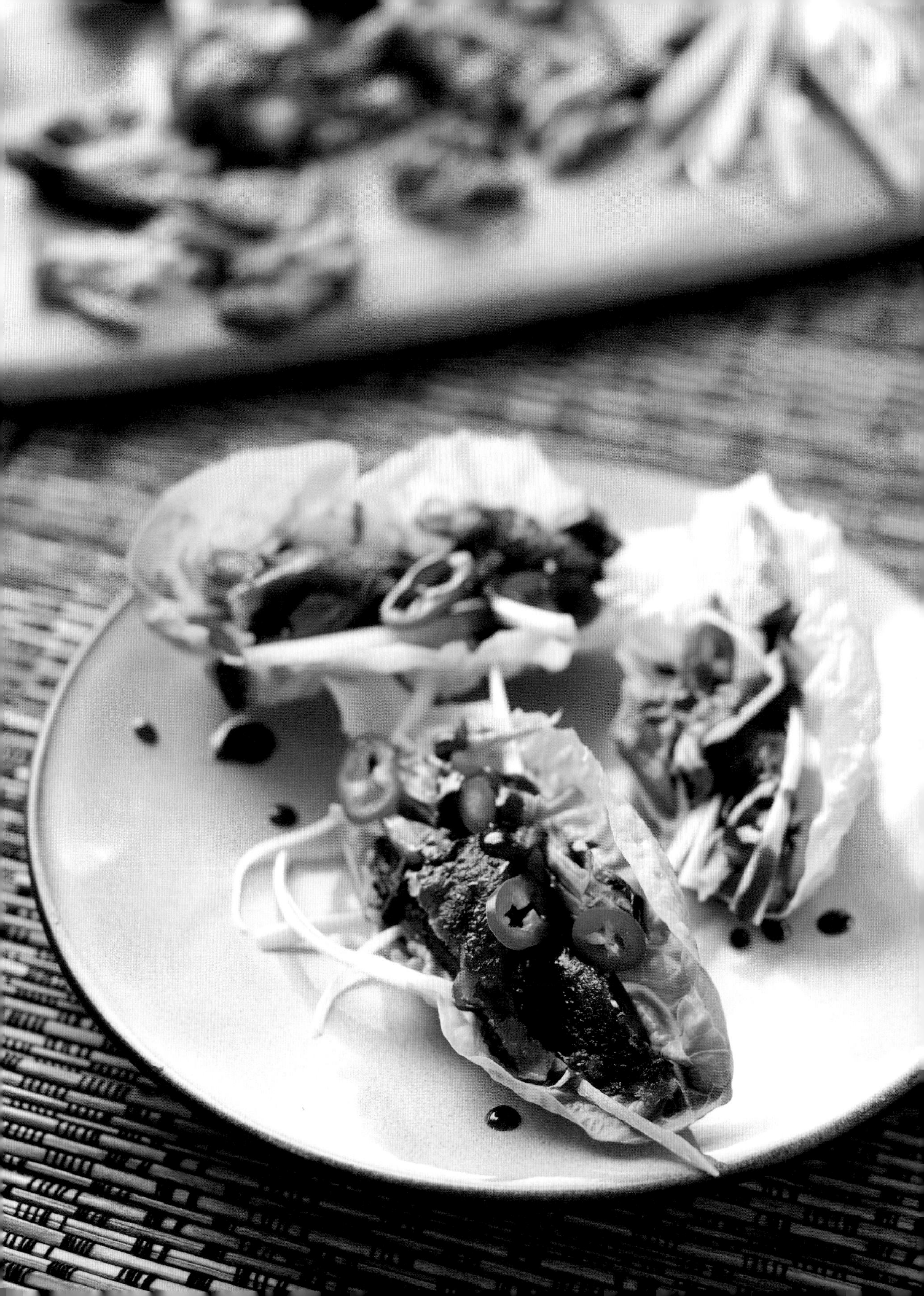

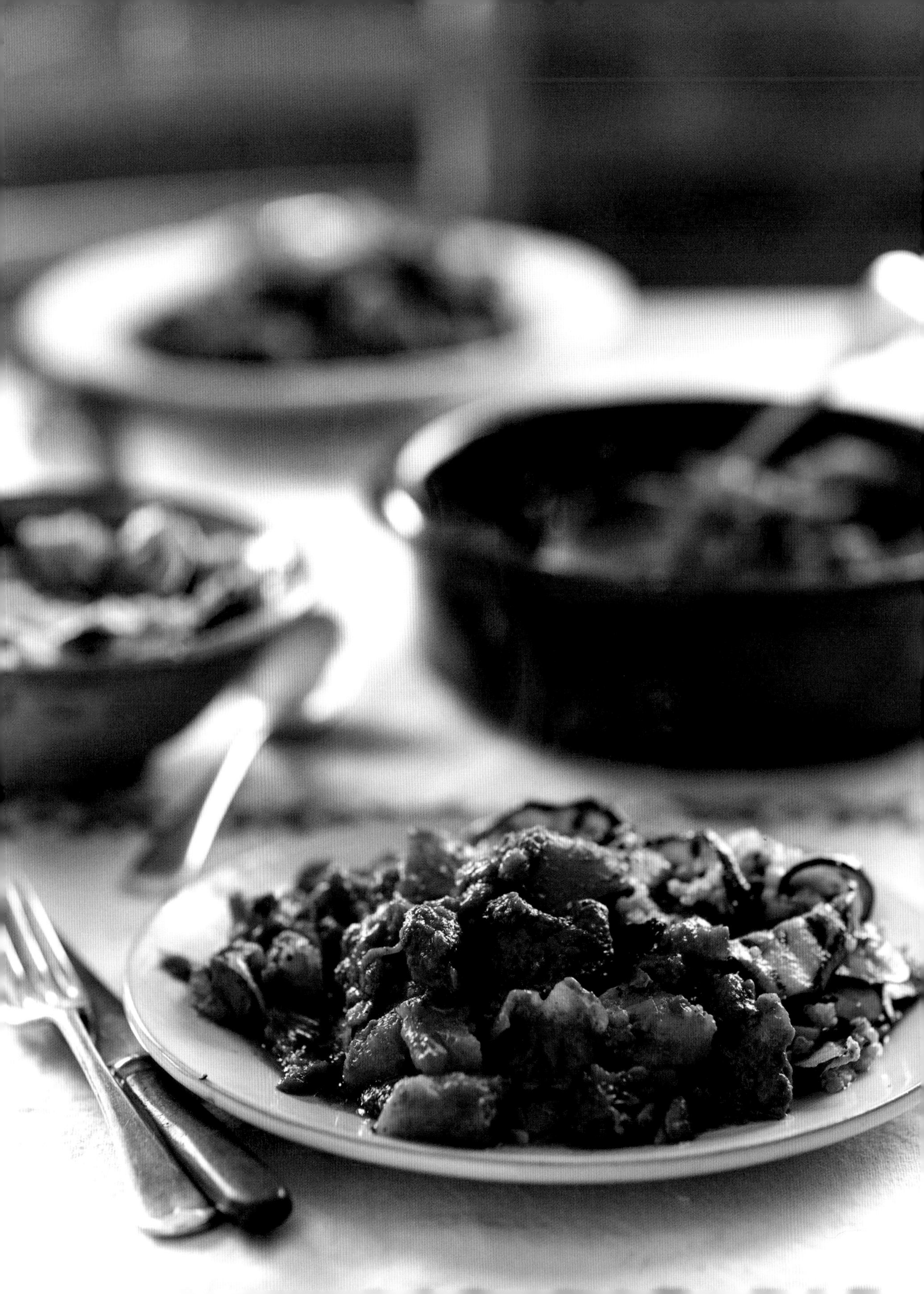

Lamb tagine

This is one of the easiest stews to make, despite the long list of ingredients. It really is a case of chuck it in and let it cook. It is full of North African flavours, the sweetness of the apricots melding deliciously with the spices and the tang of lemon.

Serves 4

400g stewing lamb, diced
2 tbsp olive oil
1 onion, diced
1 red pepper, deseeded and diced
3 garlic cloves, diced
3cm root ginger, diced
2 tsp turmeric
3 tsp paprika
2 tsp ground cumin
1 tsp ground coriander
½-1 tsp chilli flakes, fresh chilli or paste
50g dried apricots, chopped
500ml chicken or vegetable stock
200g butternut squash pieces (you can buy them ready prepared)
Juice of half a lemon

Preheat the oven to 150°C. Put all the ingredients, except the lemon juice and butternut squash, in a casserole. Cover and cook it in the oven for 2 hours, checking it occasionally and topping up the stock if necessary. Add the lemon juice and butternut squash and cook for a further 1-2 hours. Again, add extra water if it looks dry.

Before serving, add another squeeze of lemon and some salt and black pepper. Serve with quinoa (see page 99) and a green vegetable such as steamed courgettes.

- **CALORIES** 420
- PROTEIN 32G
- FAT 27G
- FIBRE 3G
- CARBS 16G

Hungarian goulash

A rich, thick beef soup from Hungary, ideal for warming up a dark wintery evening. It looks like a lot of ingredients, but it is very easy to assemble.

Serves 4

2 tbsp olive oil
2 medium onions, chopped
1 garlic clove, diced
100g baby carrots or carrots cut into batons
400g stewing steak, diced
1 green pepper and 1 red pepper, deseeded and chopped
2 tbsp paprika
1 tsp nutmeg
3 tsp mixed herbs
2 bay leaves
1 tbsp cornflour
3 tbsp tomato puree
200ml beef stock
400g tin chopped tomatoes
200ml red wine
1 tbsp Worcestershire sauce
1 tbsp cider vinegar
150ml soured cream or fromage frais
Generous handful of parsley, chopped

Preheat the oven to 150°C. Heat the oil in an ovenproof casserole and gently fry the onion, garlic and carrots till softened (about 7-8 minutes). Tip in the meat and stir to brown it all over.

Add the peppers, spices and herbs, season with salt and pepper, and cook for 2 minutes. Scatter over the cornflour and mix it in well before adding the tomato purée, stock, tomatoes, wine, Worcestershire sauce and vinegar. Bring it to a simmer, then transfer the casserole to the oven and cook for 3-4 hours, checking that it has not dried out and stirring occasionally.

Serve the goulash in a bowl with a dollop of soured cream and chopped fresh parsley. You could also serve it with roasted cauliflower (see page 165).

- **CALORIES** 350
- PROTEIN 28G
- FAT 15G
- FIBRE 3G
- CARBS 27G

Spanish chicken with chorizo and beans

Serves 2

2 tbsp olive oil
2 large or 4 small skinless, boneless chicken thighs
1 onion, chopped
2 chorizo sausages (100g), chopped
1 tsp thyme
Sprig of rosemary
2 garlic cloves, chopped
85g olives, drained
150ml chicken stock
400g tin chopped tomatoes
Juice of half a lemon
400g tin haricot or cannellini beans, drained and rinsed

Preheat the oven to 170°C. In a heavy casserole, heat 1 tbsp olive oil and brown the chicken all over. Meanwhile, in a separate pan, heat 1 tbsp olive oil and gently fry the onion, chorizo, herbs and garlic for about 5 minutes, then transfer the mixture to the main casserole. Add the olives, stock, beans, tomatoes and lemon juice and bring to the boil. Then put the lid on and place the casserole in the oven for 50-60 minutes. Serve with veg such as steamed cavolo nero or steamed or griddled courgettes.

Tip: to add extra flavour use olives stuffed with anchovies (assuming you don't get carried away like me and eat them first).

- **CALORIES** 495
- PROTEIN 38G
- FAT 19G
- FIBRE 16G
- CARBS 47G

Piri piri chicken

This is quite a spicy dish – piri piri means 'pepper pepper' in Swahili – but you can adjust how much flavouring you add, particularly if you make your own.

Serves 2

2 tbsp olive oil
1 tbsp cider vinegar
3 garlic cloves
1-2 tsp piri piri flavouring (or make your own: see tip)
2 medium-sized boneless chicken thighs
2 red peppers, deseeded and sliced
100g small tomatoes
1 fennel bulb, cut into quarters through the base
1 lime (or lemon), cut into quarters

To make the marinade, mix together the olive oil, vinegar, garlic and piri piri flavouring. Place the chicken in a large baking dish and pour the marinade over. Leave it at room temperature for 1 hour, or in the fridge for 4 hours.

Preheat the oven to 180°C. Add the red peppers, tomatoes, fennel and lime to the chicken and stir them into the marinade with some salt and a generous amount of black pepper. Bake the chicken for 40-50 minutes. Serve it with a small portion of brown rice, lentils or quinoa (2 tbsp maximum per person) and a green salad.

Tip: to make your own piri piri, mix 1 tsp paprika, 1 tsp dried oregano and 1-2 fresh chillies, seeds removed and diced (or 1-2 tsp chilli flakes).

- **CALORIES** 270
- PROTEIN 12G
- FAT 18G
- FIBRE 4G
- CARBS 13G

Coq au vin

A classic French dish made with braised chicken and a rich red wine and mushroom sauce. Served here with cauliflower mash to mop up the flavours in the gravy.

Serves 4

1 tbsp olive oil
4 chicken legs
10 shallots
50g pancetta, or smoked bacon lardons
1 garlic clove, crushed
200g chestnut mushrooms, sliced
2 tsp dried thyme
2-3 bay leaves
1 tbsp cornflour
400ml red wine
300ml chicken stock
Bouquet garni
1 carrot, cut into batons
Handful of parsley, chopped

Preheat the oven to 180°C. Heat the oil in a large ovenproof pan and fry the chicken, turning it frequently, until it is golden all over. Add the shallots, pancetta, garlic, mushrooms and herbs and let them cook gently for 5 minutes, then scatter over the cornflour. Add the wine and stock, bouquet garni and carrot and stir well. Transfer the dish to the oven and cook for 30 minutes.

If the sauce is too runny, pour some of it into a pan, bring it to the boil and let it simmer uncovered to reduce it. Scatter over the chopped parsley and serve it with cauliflower mash (see page 196).

- **CALORIES** 510
- PROTEIN 40G
- FAT 28G
- FIBRE 2G
- CARBS 10G

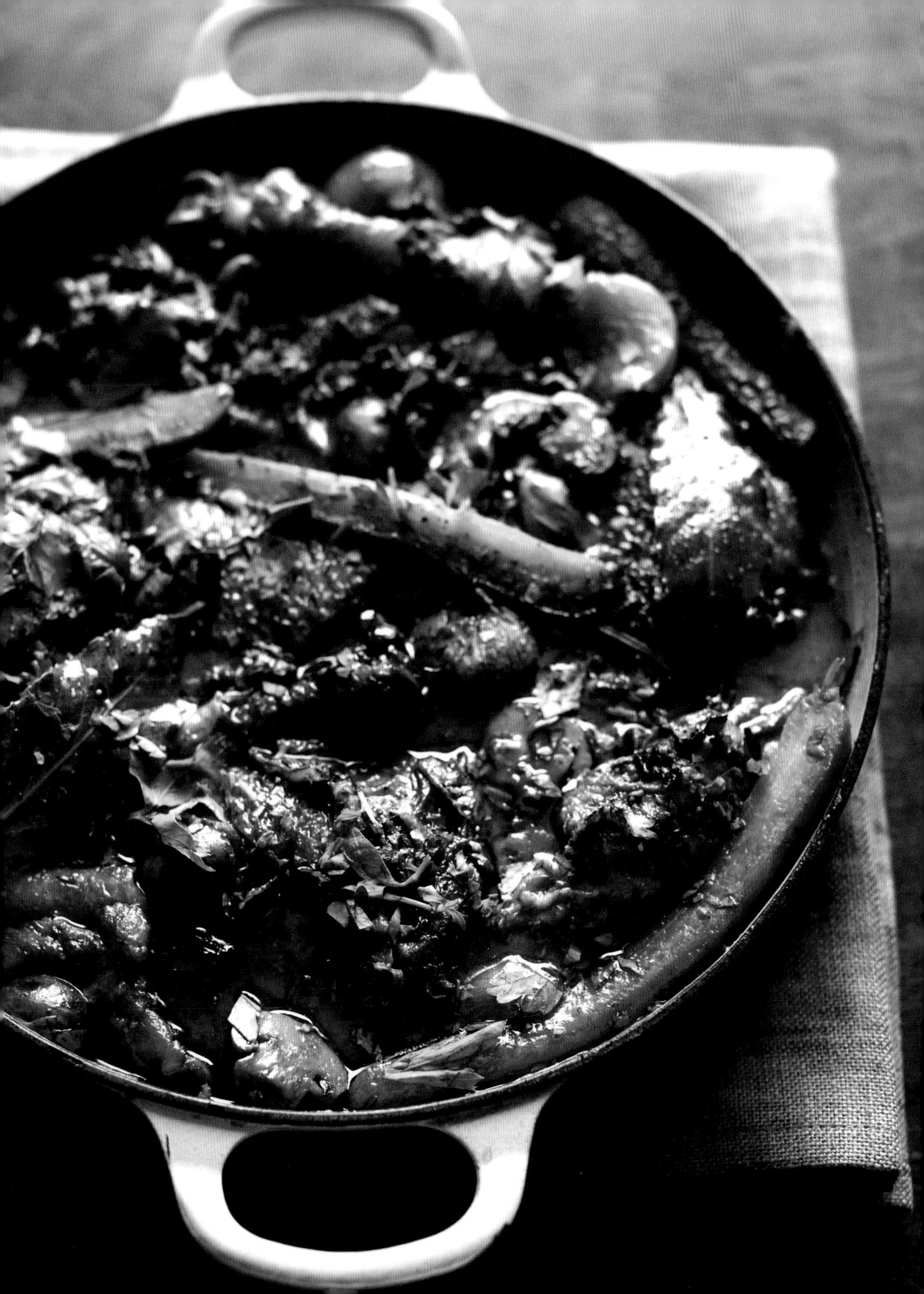

Skinny cottage pie

Perfect comfort food. Swapping the starchy mashed potato topping for cauliflower mash makes all the difference.

Serves 6

1 tbsp olive oil
1 small onion, diced
450-500g minced beef
2 garlic cloves, sliced
1-2 tsp dried thyme
400g tin chopped tomatoes
1 beef or vegetable stock cube or 1 tsp Worcestershire sauce
2 carrots, diced
2 bay leaves

For the cauliflower mash:
1 medium cauliflower
75g Cheddar, grated
2 tsp olive oil
2 tbsp full-fat fromage frais
2 spring onions, finely chopped
1 tsp Parmesan, grated

Preheat the oven to 200°C. Heat the olive oil in a saucepan and sweat the onion till it is golden, then add the beef, garlic and thyme. When the meat is cooked through, stir in the tomatoes, stock cube (or Worcestershire sauce), carrots, bay leaves and enough water to cover the mixture. Put the lid on and simmer for about an hour.

Meanwhile, to make the mash, chop the cauliflower into pieces about 2cm in diameter, then steam or boil them for 8-10 minutes or until they are soft. Mash the cauliflower vigorously. Note that it won't form the creamy solid texture of mashed potatoes). Add the grated cheese, olive oil, fromage frais and spring onions and mix well.

Put the mince in an ovenproof dish, dollop the mash on top, then scatter over the Parmesan. Bake the pie on the middle shelf of the oven for 20-30 minutes or until it is crispy on top.

Tips: to meld the flavours, boil the mince gently for an hour if you have time, stirring and topping up with water or stock as needed. To improve the texture of the mash, you can add half a tin of chickpeas (drained and rinsed first). This will add 150 calories to the dish.

- **CALORIES** 310
- PROTEIN 23G
- FAT 21G
- FIBRE 3G
- CARBS 8G

Creamy fish bake

Serves 6

1 tbsp olive oil
4 shallots (or 2 small onions), chopped
3 garlic cloves, crushed
25g butter
200ml double cream
1 tbsp crème fraîche
1 tbsp chives (or spring onion), finely chopped
1 tbsp parsley, finely chopped
1 tbsp tarragon, finely chopped (or 1 tsp dried)
50ml white wine
1 tbsp lemon juice
2-3 eggs
1 small celeriac, peeled and chopped
400g mixed fish (e.g. haddock, cod and smoked salmon), cut into chunks
50g Cheddar, grated

Preheat the oven to 200°C. Heat the oil in a frying pan and gently cook the shallots and garlic for 4-5 minutes or until they have softened. In a separate pan, melt half the butter, then pour in the cream and crème fraîche and heat the mixture without letting it boil. Add the shallots and garlic together with the herbs, followed by the white wine. Season the sauce with a pinch of salt and pepper, and lemon juice to taste.

Meanwhile, boil the eggs in a pan of water for 6-7 minutes, then plunge them into cold water to cool them. Peel and roughly chop them before stirring them into the sauce. Place the celeriac in a pan of boiling water and cook it for 6-8 minutes or until it is tender, then mash it with the remaining butter.

Stir the fish pieces into the sauce and bring it to the boil, then transfer the mixture to an ovenproof dish, and spread the mash over the top. Sprinkle with the grated cheese and bake it in the oven for around 15 minutes.

- **CALORIES** 360
- PROTEIN 19G
- FAT 29G
- FIBRE 3G
- CARBS 3G

Skinny aubergine 'lasagne'

Inspired by a great recipe from Cherianne on the Blood Sugar Diet website in which we use thinly sliced aubergine instead of courgette as it keeps its texture better. An excellent low-cal, low-carb Mediterranean-style vegetarian meal for anyone missing pasta.

Serves 4

50g raw spinach (or defrosted frozen spinach), chopped
50g Parmesan, grated
100g cottage cheese (or ricotta, but note it has more calories and less protein)
½ red pepper, deseeded and finely chopped
200g mushrooms, chopped
1 fat garlic clove, crushed
2 tsp dried oregano
1 tsp dried basil
300ml passata
1 tbsp olive oil
200g aubergine, sliced lengthwise in ½cm strips
12 cherry tomatoes, halved, or 6 larger tomatoes, chopped
50g Cheddar, grated

Preheat the oven to 200°C. Finely chop the spinach and mix it with the Parmesan and cottage cheese in a bowl, and season to taste. Place the chopped red pepper and mushrooms in a separate bowl along with the garlic, herbs, passata and olive oil. Season well.

Spread half of the tomato and veg mixture over the bottom of a rectangular ovenproof dish or tin, followed by alternating layers of sliced aubergines and the cheese and spinach mix. The last layer should be aubergines. Pour the rest of the tomato mix over the top and dot with the cherry tomatoes. Cover the dish with foil and bake it for approximately 30 minutes or until the aubergine feels soft and thoroughly cooked.

Remove the foil and sprinkle grated cheese over the top of the lasagne. Put it back in the oven for another 10-15 minutes or until the cheese has melted and browned. Serve with a crunchy green salad.

Tip: you could add Quorn or minced meat to the tomato mix if desired.

- **CALORIES** 200
- PROTEIN 14G
- FAT 13G
- FIBRE 3G
- CARBS 7G

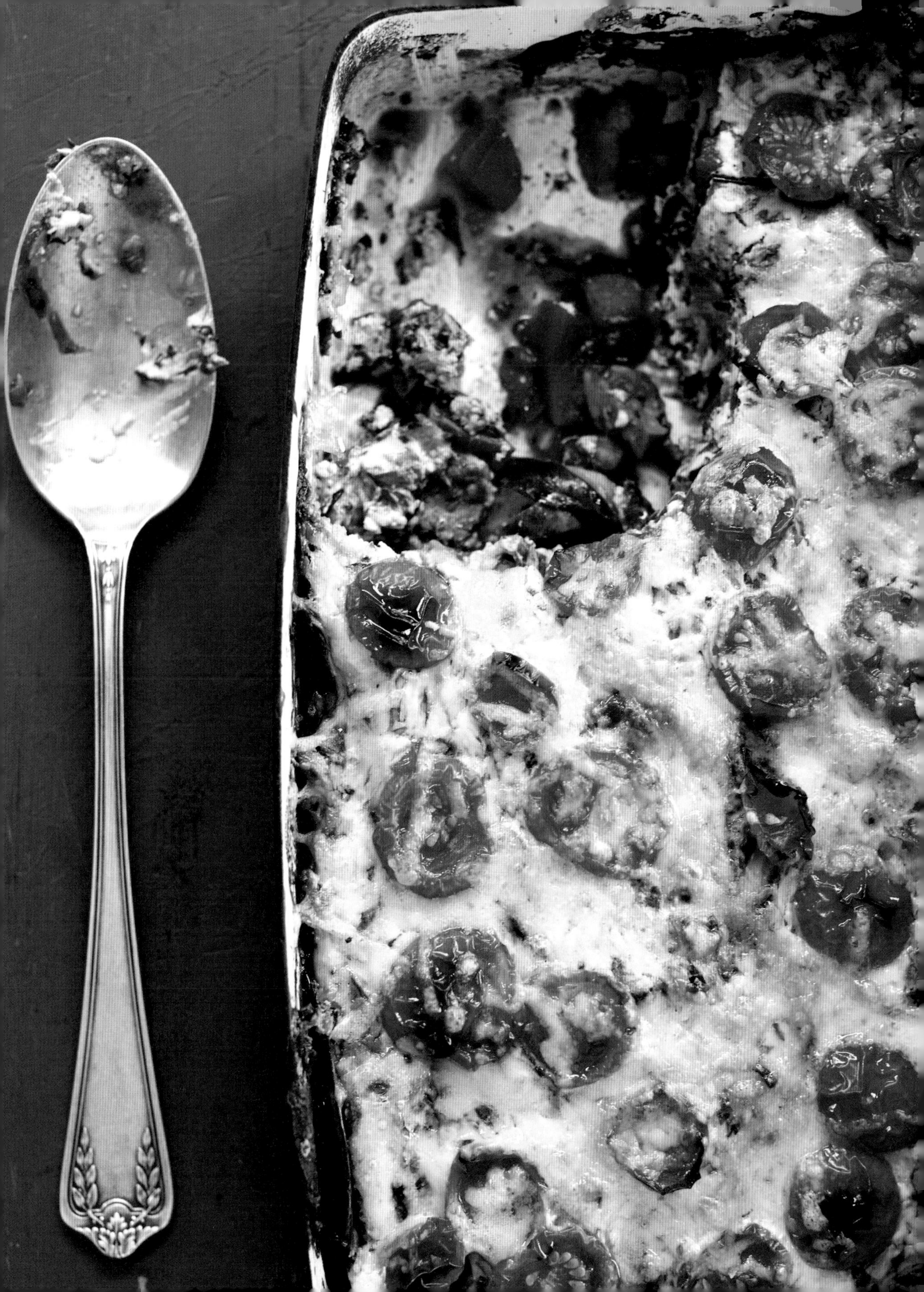

Chicken and mushroom 'pie'

A scrummy meal in one dish, just without the pastry.

Serves 6

2 small onions, diced
2 tbsp olive oil
8 boneless chicken thighs (or 6 medium-sized chicken breasts), cut into chunks
200g mushrooms, sliced
½ tsp ground nutmeg
1 level tbsp cornflour
100ml chicken stock (made with ¼ stock cube)
2 heaped tbsp crème fraîche
2 tsp mustard
1 tsp dried tarragon (or 2 bay leaves)

For the topping:
Outer leaves of a large white cabbage
1 small cauliflower, broken into florets
2 large leeks, diced into 1-2cm pieces (discard green ends)
50 g Parmesan, grated
1-2 tsp paprika

Preheat the oven to 180°C. Gently fry the onions in 1 tbsp olive oil in a deep metal pie tray over the hob – a nice trick for saving washing-up from Jamie Oliver (or use a saucepan and transfer the contents to the dish later).

When the onions have softened, add the chicken and cook it until it is slightly browned, then stir in the mushrooms and nutmeg. Fry gently for a few more minutes. Scatter the cornflour over the onions and chicken and mix it into the juices. Then pour in the chicken stock and the crème fraîche along with the mustard and tarragon (or bay leaves) and some seasoning. Stir and simmer gently for a few minutes.

Meanwhile, prepare the topping by cutting each cabbage leaf in half with a sharp knife and removing the tough central stalk, then laying the leaves on top of the chicken and mushroom sauce, slightly overlapping so it cooks without drying out. Mix the cauliflower and leeks in a bowl with the rest of the olive oil and season well. Spread this mixture over the layer of cabbage, scatter the Parmesan and then the paprika on top and bake the pie in the oven for about 30 minutes, checking after about 20 minutes. Serve with green vegetables.

Tip: chicken thighs tend to have more flavour and are also cheaper than breast.

- **CALORIES** 250
- PROTEIN 26G
- FAT 12G
- FIBRE 3G
- CARBS 9G

Low-carb lamb hotpot

A classic Lancashire hotpot topped with butternut squash. This benefits from several hours of cooking so the meat melts in your mouth.

Serves 4

2 tbsp olive oil
400g lamb, diced
2 onions, chopped
½ tsp dried thyme
Sprig of rosemary
4 carrots, cut into batons
2 tsp cornflour
500ml lamb or chicken stock
½ tsp black peppercorns
1 tbsp Worcestershire sauce
1 butternut squash, peeled, halved and sliced into 3-5cm semi-circles
50g Parmesan, grated

Preheat the oven to 170°C. Heat 1 tbsp oil in a medium-sized heavy casserole dish with a lid. Add the lamb and, when it is starting to brown, stir in the diced onions and cook gently for a few minutes. Add the thyme, rosemary and carrots and mix the cornflour into the juices. Pour in the Worcestershire sauce and enough stock to cover the meat, along with the peppercorns. Stir well, cover the dish and place it in the oven.

After about an hour, check that it has not dried out and if necessary add water. Then cover the surface with an overlapping layer of butternut squash slices. Drizzle with the remaining olive oil, replace the lid and return it to the oven.

After half an hour, check once again that it is not drying out (you may need to add half a cup or so of water – if so, tip this in round the edges so the top doesn't go soggy). Then scatter the Parmesan on the surface, and cook the hotpot for another hour, until the top is golden brown. Serve with dark green veg such as cavolo nero or kale.

Tip: you can use celeriac instead of butternut squash if you prefer.

- **CALORIES** 380
- PROTEIN 27G
- FAT 20G
- FIBRE 5G
- CARBS 23G

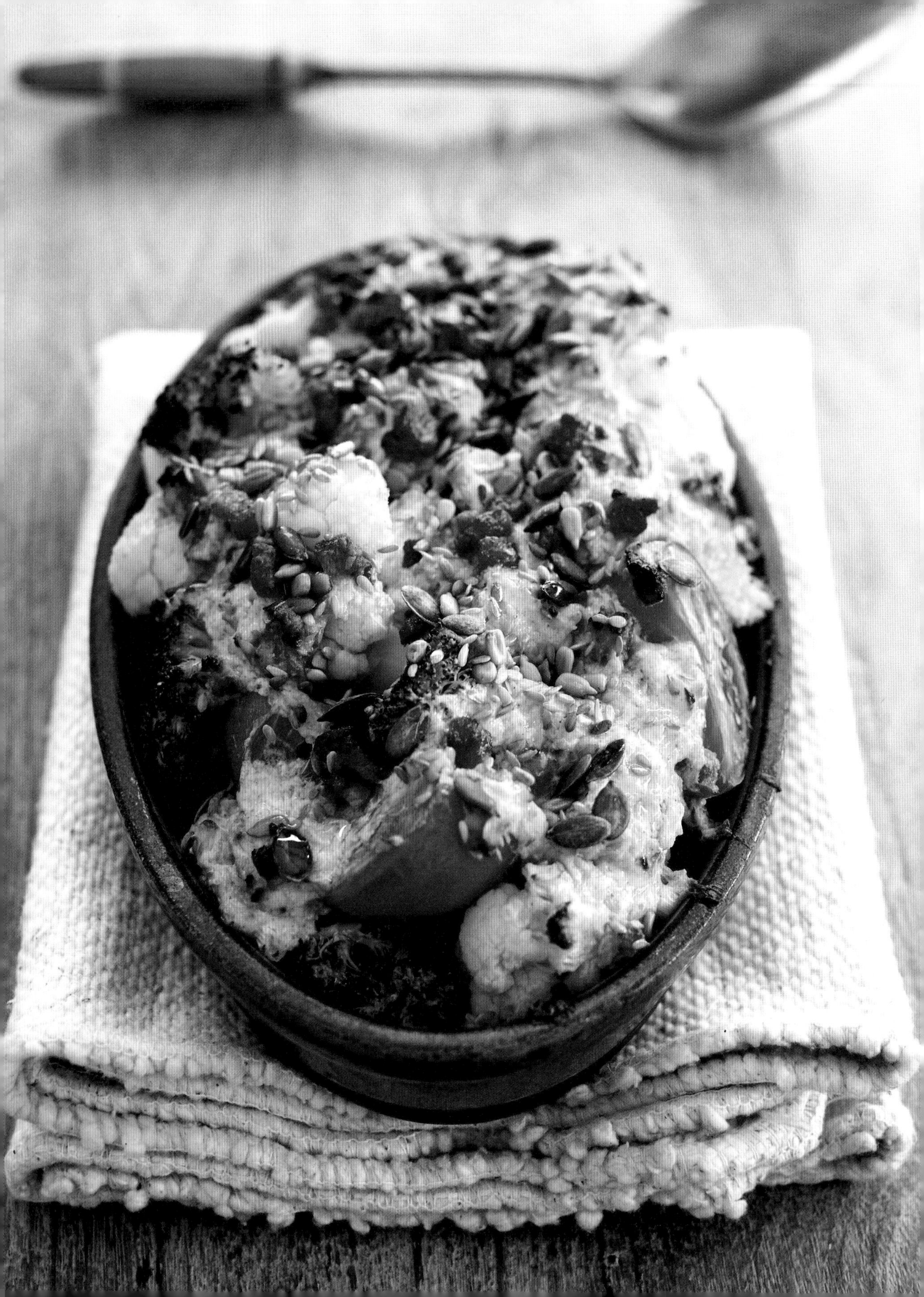

Pancetta, broccoli and tomato gratin

Serves 4

1 head each of broccoli and cauliflower
100g pancetta
Drizzle of olive oil
100g soft cheese
50g Cheddar, grated
1 tsp mustard
100g soured cream
2 spring onions, finely chopped
½ tsp cayenne pepper
2 large tomatoes, sliced
3 tbsp Parmesan, grated
3 tbsp mixed seeds (e.g. Munchy seeds)

Preheat the oven to 180°C. Cut the cauliflower and broccoli into small florets and steam them until they are tender but still crisp – about 4-5 minutes. Drain them well and place them in a greased shallow baking dish.

Meanwhile, fry the pancetta in a drizzle of olive oil. In a bowl, mix together the soft cheese, soured cream, Cheddar, mustard, spring onions and cayenne pepper and season well with salt and pepper. Spread this mixture over the cauliflower and broccoli as evenly as possible. Lay the tomatoes on top of the veg and sprinkle the Parmesan and seeds over the surface. Bake the gratin for 20 minutes or until the topping is golden brown and bubbling.

- **CALORIES** 340
- PROTEIN 22G
- FAT 23G
- FIBRE 4G
- CARBS 10G

Baked fish and chorizo parcels

Serves 2

1 tbsp olive oil plus extra for drizzling
1 fennel bulb, cut into strips
1 chorizo sausage, diced
2 thick cod steaks
50g cherry tomatoes, each pierced with a sharp knife
Handful of basil leaves
2 tbsp cider vinegar

Preheat the oven to 190°C. Heat the oil in a pan and fry the fennel and chorizo for 3-4 minutes.

Take 2 square sheets of foil and pile half the fennel mixture in the middle of each one. Place the cod on top, drizzle it with olive oil and season it well with salt and pepper. Then add the cherry tomatoes and basil leaves, sprinkle on the vinegar and scrunch up the foil tightly to make a well-sealed but loose parcel. Bake the parcels in the oven for about 15 minutes and serve with salad or steamed thin green beans.

Tip: you could use anchovies instead of chorizo. Drape 2-3 fillets over each piece of cod before you put it in the oven.

- **CALORIES** 270
- PROTEIN 33G
- FAT 15G
- FIBRE 1G
- CARBS 2G

Gammon steak with red cabbage

The rich, sweet-tasting red cabbage works really well with the salty meat.

Serves 2

3 tbsp olive oil
1 onion, diced
½ small red cabbage, outer leaves removed, quartered, cored and finely sliced
150ml vegetable stock
2 tart eating apples (such as Braeburn, Cox or Granny Smith), diced into 2cm pieces
½ tsp cumin seeds or ¼ tsp ground allspice
2 gammon steaks, trimmed of fat (or 2 pork chops)
4 tbsp balsamic vinegar
1 tbsp crème fraîche
Handful of parsley or chives

Preheat the oven to 170°C. On a low heat, sweat the onion in 2 tbsp olive oil in an ovenproof casserole until it starts to caramelise. Then add the cabbage and continue to cook for a few more minutes. Add the stock, balsamic vinegar, apples, cumin seeds, a pinch of salt and freshly ground black pepper. Cover and cook in the oven for 1 hour, stirring occasionally and adding a little water if required.

Heat the rest of the olive oil in a frying pan and fry the gammon steaks on both sides. Season them with black pepper. Serve with roasted cauliflower (see page 165). Put a dollop of crème fraîche on top of the cabbage mixture and garnish with parsley or chives

- **CALORIES** 420
- PROTEIN 19G
- FAT 31G
- FIBRE 4G
- CARBS 16G

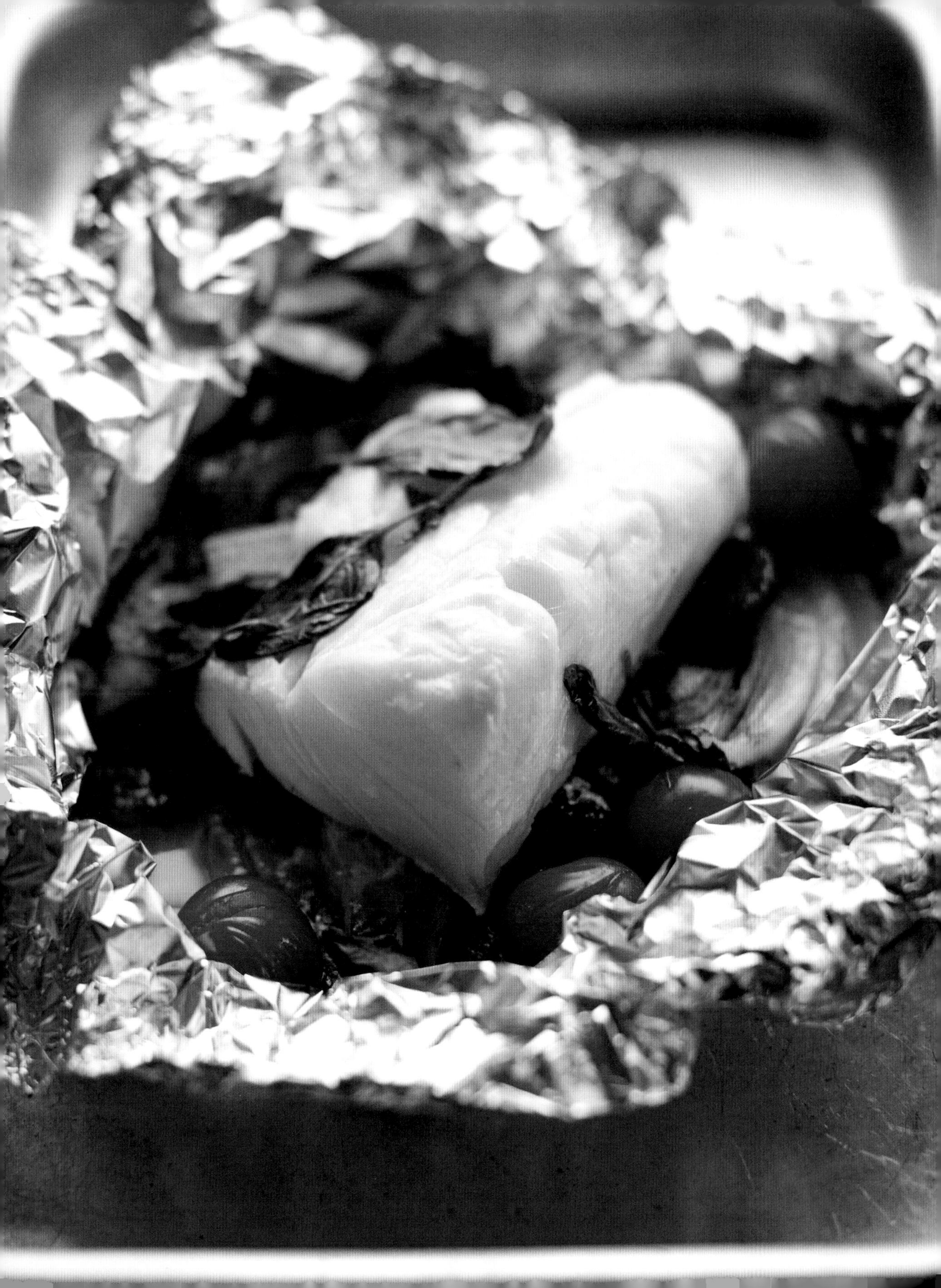

Lazy chicken and spicy lentils

This delicious dish, originally from the Caribbean, is super-easy to prepare. We have replaced the rice with lentils and love their slightly chewy, nutty taste.

Serves 4

Juice of 2 limes
3 garlic cloves, crushed
1 tsp chilli flakes
1 tsp dried thyme
2 tbsp light olive oil
4 chicken thighs with skin (ideally boneless)
1 onion, chopped
200g chestnut mushrooms, chopped
160g dried green lentils (or a 400g tin green lentils, drained and rinsed to add later on)
200ml chicken stock (reduce to 100ml if using tinned lentils)

Combine the lime juice, garlic, chilli flakes and thyme in a bowl to make a marinade. Season it with pepper and salt and toss the chicken in it. Cover the bowl and leave it at room temperature for 2 hours or in the fridge overnight.

Preheat the oven to 180°C. Then brown the chicken on both sides in 1 tbsp oil in a large frying pan. Scatter the onion and mushrooms over the base of a deep ovenproof dish. Add the dried lentils, place the chicken pieces on top skin side up and drizzle with the rest of the oil. Prepare 200ml of stock in the bowl containing the remaining marinade juices and pour it over the chicken and veg. Cover the dish and place it in the oven.

After 20 minutes check it and add more stock (or some water) if it's looking dry. Cook for about 20 minutes more with the lid off (add the tinned lentils at this stage if using). Serve with green veg or a salad.

- CALORIES 460
- PROTEIN 52G
- FAT 29G
- FIBRE 10G
- CARBS 52G

Michael's easy roast chicken with garlic and thyme

Roasts probably don't come to mind when you think about diet food. But a roast without the starchy potatoes or parsnips can be just that.

Serves 6

3-4 garlic cloves
Large knob of butter
2 tsp dried thyme or tarragon (sprigs of fresh even better)
1 large free-range chicken
1 lemon
1 onion, halved
400g whole baby carrots or carrots cut into batons
1 large cauliflower, broken into florets
1 tbsp olive oil
400g green veg

For the gravy:
1 tbsp cornflour
1 chicken stock cube + 300ml hot water
½ tbsp soy sauce

Preheat the oven to 200°C. Mash the garlic with the butter and herbs in a small bowl. Place the chicken in a large roasting tray. Cut a few holes in the skin over the breasts and thighs, and push blobs of the garlic butter under it. Also smear some over the rest of the chicken skin and season well.

Squeeze the lemon juice over the whole chicken, rubbing it in, and put the rind inside the cavity. Add the onion halves to the tray cut side downwards. Roast the chicken in the oven, allowing 20 minutes per pound plus 20 minutes extra. Baste it every 15-20 minutes. Add the carrots to the roasting tray about 40 minutes before the end of cooking time.

Place the cauliflower florets on a separate roasting tray. Season them, drizzle over the olive oil and bake them at the top of the oven for about 25 minutes. Also prepare the green veg, such as thin green beans or runner beans, so they are ready to boil or steam while you make the gravy.

When the chicken is cooked, remove it to a carving block and let it rest. The onion can be eaten or discarded if charred. Stir the cornflour into the oils and juices in the roasting tray, before adding 300ml water, the stock cube and the soy sauce, and continue to stir over a gentle heat until the gravy has thickened. Pour it into a warmed jug when you are ready to serve.

Tips: the onion in the baking tray caramelises and produces sweet tangy juices for a perfect gravy. Use any leftover chicken in a soup, a stir-fry or bulgar wheat risotto (see page 129).

- **CALORIES** 260
- PROTEIN 28G
- FAT 15G
- FIBRE 4G
- CARBS 17G

Veg Sides

We all need to eat more vegetables, whether we are on the Blood Sugar Diet or not. And you will find that on 800 calories a day they become a lifeline – filling you up and providing vital flavour, texture and crunch. To help you reap the benefits of their huge range of health-promoting nutrients, we suggest you aim to fill half your plate at any main meal with non-starchy vegetables. These will give you a slow-release form of energy with little impact on blood sugars.

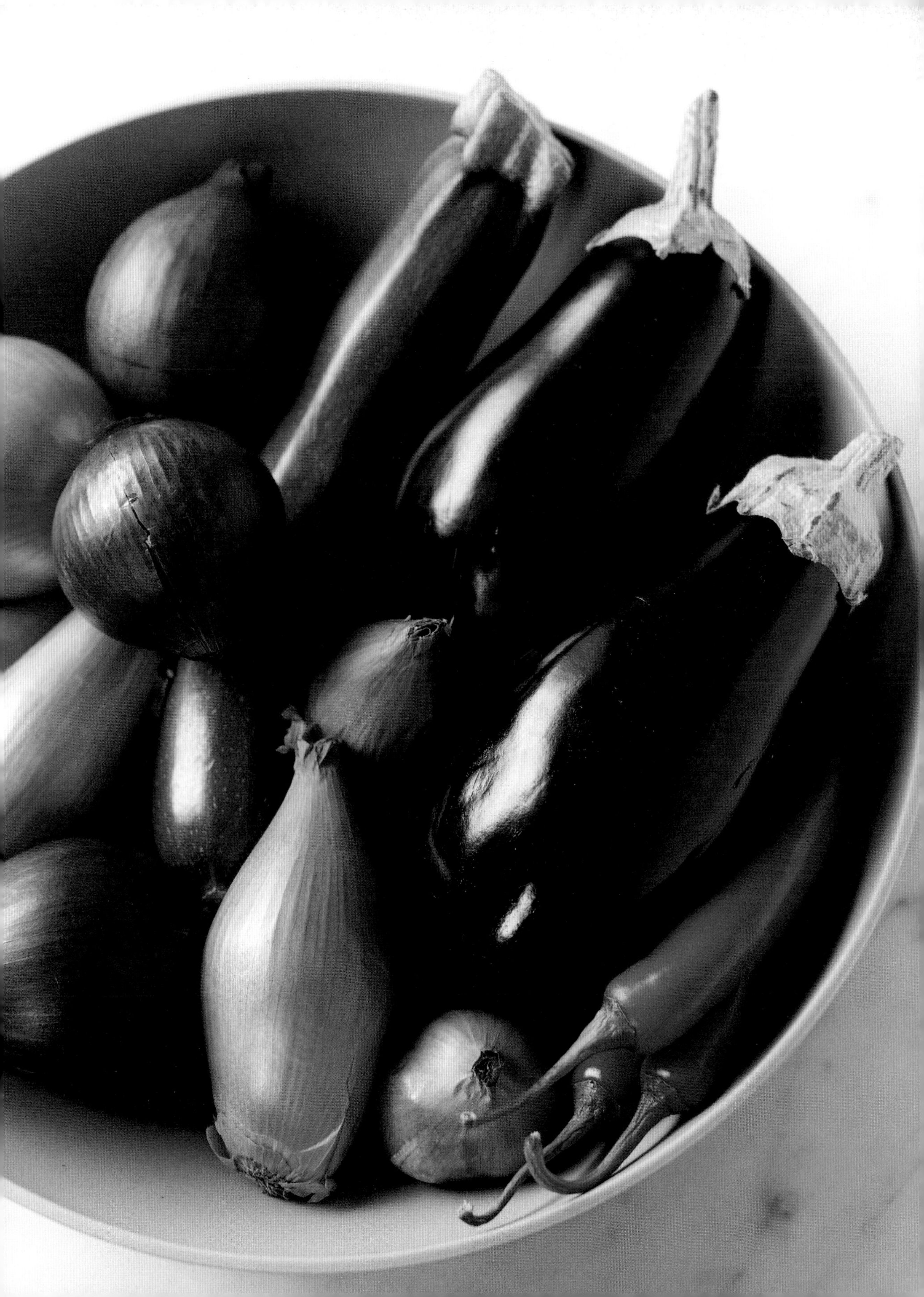

Simple salads

These make excellent side salads, but you can also add extras such as cheese, nuts, seeds, tofu or smoked fish to turn them into a meal in themselves.

Mixed leaf salad with rocket and shaved Parmesan

You can't go wrong with this Mediterranean classic, which takes only a few minutes to prepare and goes with almost anything.

Serves 2

1 bag of rocket or mixed leaves
1 tbsp olive oil
½ tbsp balsamic vinegar
30g Parmesan, shaved

Place the salad leaves in the bowl, drizzle over the olive oil and vinegar with a pinch of salt and some freshly ground black pepper, then scatter the Parmesan on top.

- **CALORIES** 120
- PROTEIN 7G
- FAT 10G
- FIBRE 1G
- CARBS 0G

Crunchy red coleslaw

This colourful crunchy coleslaw goes particularly well with cold meats.

Serves 4

½ small red cabbage, very finely sliced
1 fennel bulb, finely sliced
1 small red onion, finely sliced
1 carrot, grated
2 tbsp pomegranate seeds (or 1 small red apple, grated)
2 tbsp each mayonnaise and Greek yoghurt, blended together
1 tbsp chopped walnuts, toasted (or 2 tsp chia seeds)

Mix the vegetables together in a bowl, stir in the mayo and yoghurt dressing with a pinch of salt and some freshly ground black pepper, and scatter the nuts or seeds on top.

- **CALORIES** 120
- PROTEIN 3G
- FAT 9G
- FIBRE 3G
- CARBS 7G

Tabbouleh with pine nuts

As with traditional tabbouleh recipes, relatively little bulgar wheat is used; it's really more of a parsley salad, which makes it an even less carb-rich addition to a meal.

Serves 4

50g bulgar wheat
75g parsley, coarsely chopped
25g mint leaves, coarsely chopped
50g tomatoes, deseeded and finely diced
50g cucumber, deseeded and finely diced
1 spring onion (or 1 tbsp red onion), finely sliced
50g pine nuts, toasted and coarsely chopped
Handful of pomegranate seeds (or raisins)

For the dressing:
1 garlic clove, crushed
2 tbsp lemon juice
3 tbsp olive oil
1 tsp cumin seeds
½ tsp ground cinnamon
½ tsp cayenne pepper

Put the bulgar wheat in a small saucepan and cover it with 1-2cm stock. Bring it to the boil, then reduce the heat and simmer gently for 10 minutes, adding a splash more water if necessary. Turn off the heat and let it steam, covered, for a further 10-15 minutes.

Meanwhile, make the dressing by whisking all the ingredients together in a small bowl with some salt and freshly ground black pepper.

Mix all the vegetables, the pine nuts and herbs together in a bowl. When the bulgar wheat has cooled, add it to the salad and stir in the dressing before scattering over the pomegranate seeds.

Tip: toasting pine nuts brings out the flavour – simply put them in a dry frying pan over a medium to high heat, shaking and stirring intermittently for a few minutes until they are golden brown.

- **CALORIES** 150
- PROTEIN 4G
- FAT 9G
- FIBRE 2G
- CARBS 13G

Broccoli and asparagus salad

The creamy, tangy buttermilk dressing here really brings this salad to life. Buttermilk contains healthy live bacteria which are good for your gut, while the broccoli is rich in antioxidants which mop up damaging free radicals.

Serves 4

1 head of broccoli
1 large bunch of asparagus (about 12 stems)
Buttermilk dressing (see page 176)
20g flaked almonds

Break the broccoli into small florets and cut the asparagus into 3-4cm lengths. If the asparagus is thick, slice it lengthwise first. Put the vegetables in a large bowl and drizzle the buttermilk dressing over. Toast the flaked almonds in a small dry frying pan for 1-2 minutes (watch closely as they burn quickly), then scatter them over the salad.

Tip: if you prefer your broccoli and asparagus a bit softer you can sear it briefly on the griddle first.

- CALORIES 60
- PROTEIN 5G
- FAT 4G
- FIBRE 3G
- CARBS 2G

Spiced purple veg

Delicious hot or cold, this dish livens up almost any meal. There is evidence of lots of health benefits from eating beetroot, including lowering blood pressure, reducing the risk of heart disease and dementia, and improving muscle pains after exercise.

Serves 4

2 medium-sized beetroot, peeled
1 large red onion, sliced
½ small red cabbage, core removed, finely sliced
3 tbsp balsamic or cider vinegar
½ tsp cumin seeds
½ tsp coriander seeds
½ tsp red chilli, deseeded and finely diced (or ½ tsp chilli flakes)
1 tbsp table salt

Chop the beetroot into 2cm cubes and place it in a colander. Then add layers of onion and red cabbage, sprinkling salt between each as you go. Leave the colander over a bowl to drain for about 20 minutes.

Preheat the oven to 170°C. Rinse and drain the salted vegetables over the sink. Then place all the vegetables in a baking dish, pour over the vinegar, scatter the spices and mix together along with a pinch salt and freshly ground black pepper on top. Cover the dish with foil and bake for 30 minutes, turning the vegetables once. Serve hot or cold.

- CALORIES 40
- PROTEIN 2G
- FAT 0G
- FIBRE 3G
- CARBS 9G

Pickled cabbage (kimchi)

It is now recognised that pickling food in vinegar provides health benefits, lowering blood sugars and boosting your gut bacteria.

½ small white cabbage or Chinese cabbage, core and outer leaves removed
2 garlic cloves, finely chopped
2cm root ginger, finely chopped or grated
1 tbsp mirin (or cider vinegar)
1 tbsp Thai fish sauce (or soy sauce)
2 tsp sweet chilli sauce (see page 175), or 1-2 tsp chilli flakes and 1 tsp hoisin plum sauce
2 spring onions, finely chopped
1 tsp maple syrup (or honey)
¼ tsp salt

Finely slice the cabbage and steam or microwave it for 2 minutes. Then place it in a large jar with a lid or in a covered bowl. Meanwhile, make the marinade by mixing the rest of the ingredients in a bowl. Pour the marinade over the cabbage, mix it well and ideally leave it for up to 6 hours, but for a minimum of 30 minutes, stirring occasionally.

- **CALORIES** 80
- PROTEIN 4G
- FAT 1G
- FIBRE 3G
- CARBS 14G

Rainbow salad

I encourage my patients to eat not only more, but also different coloured vegetables. As well as making food look more enticing, the different colours represent different phytochemicals, substances which plants produce to protect themselves against bacteria, viruses, and so on, and which are also good for our health.

Serves 2

2 large handfuls of watercress
1 carrot, grated
1 pickled beetroot, diced
1 yellow pepper, deseeded and cut into strips
8 cherry tomatoes, halved
4 radishes, finely sliced
Handful of blueberries

Put all the salad ingredients in a large bowl and toss them in French vinaigrette (see page 173).

Tip: most supermarkets sell pickled beetroot.

- CALORIES 120
- PROTEIN 3G
- FAT 1G
- FIBRE 4G
- CARBS 11G

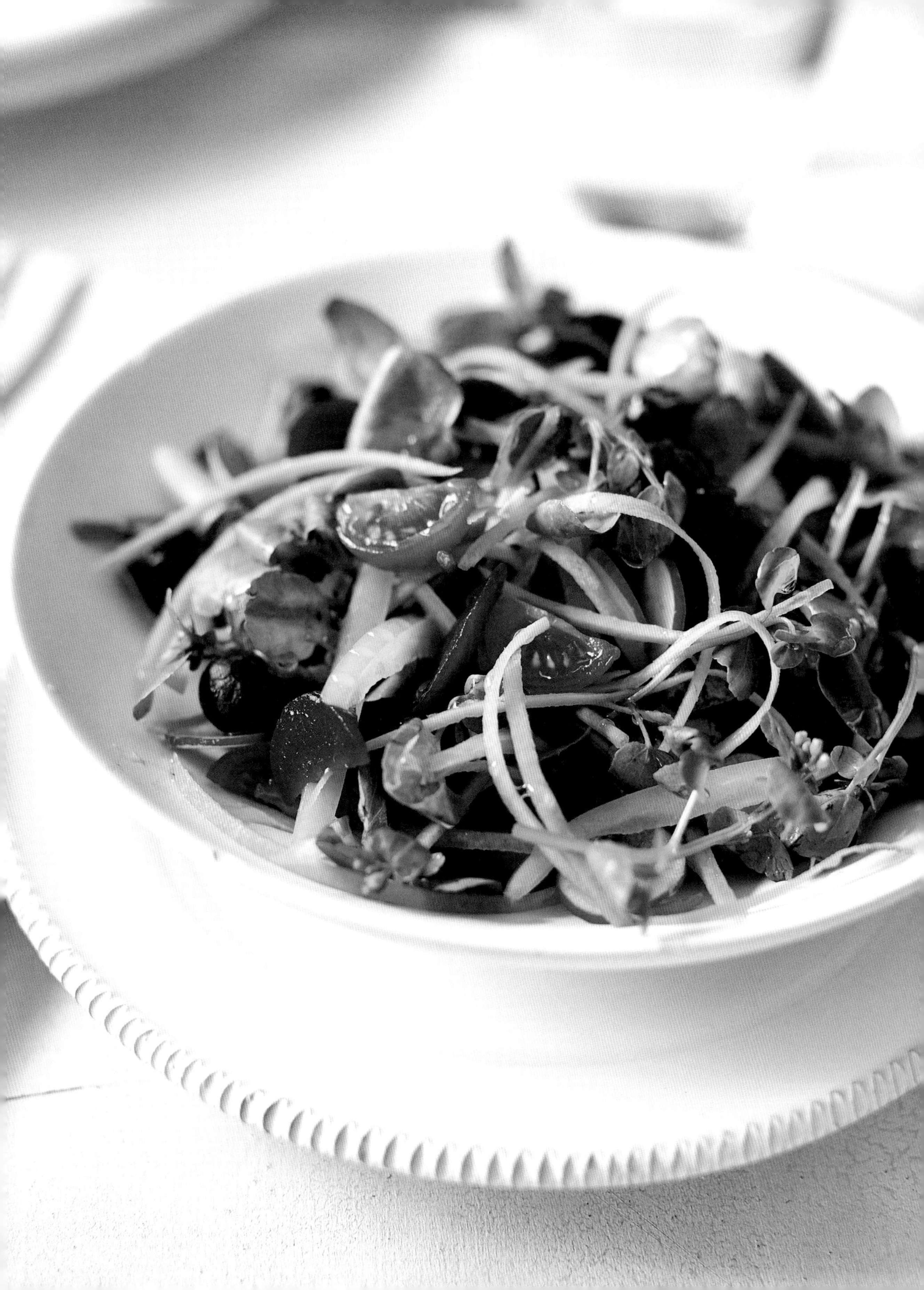

Cooked veg sides

Roasted garlicky aubergine mash

This dish is a faster and easier version of the Middle Eastern classic baba ganoush in which aubergines are charred on a grill, producing a wonderful smoky flavour. It works brilliantly as a side dish or it can be eaten as a dip with veg sticks, as a lighter alternative to hummus.

Serves 4

2 aubergines
2 tbsp olive oil
1 onion, finely diced
2 garlic cloves, crushed
½ tbsp balsamic vinegar
½ tsp fresh chilli, deseeded and finely diced (or ½ tsp chilli flakes) to taste
Handful of parsley, chopped
1 tbsp pomegranate seeds (optional)

- CALORIES 90
- PROTEIN 1G
- FAT 7G
- FIBRE 2G
- CARBS 5G

There are several ways to roast the aubergines. We do it in our old iron wok, with the heat high and the lid on. It takes about 5 minutes and there's no mess. Place the aubergines in the hot dry wok, stalks still on, and cover. To get the flavour, the skin has to burn so allow it to thicken and char before you turn it. You don't need to char it all but aim to do at least half.

Meanwhile, heat the oil in a medium-sized saucepan with a lid and sweat the onions for about 5 minutes, then stir in the garlic.

When the aubergines are sufficiently charred, remove them to a plate and allow them to cool a bit. Or if you're in a hurry, have a glass of cold water nearby to cool your fingers as you prepare them. Chop off the stalks and peel off the skin, then dice the flesh and add it to the pan. Stir in the balsamic vinegar and chilli.

Cook gently for 10-15 minutes, with the lid on, stirring occasionally. Add 1 tbsp water if it is drying out to maintain a thick creamy texture. Season and serve with parsley and pomegranate seeds, if using, scattered over.

Tips: there are other ways to char the aubergine skin. You can hold it in tongs directly over a hot flame on a gas hob (but this can be messy, when the skin bursts and juice drips everywhere); or place it under a hot grill, piercing the skin first, and turning it several times.

Cauliflower 2 ways

Having barely eaten cauliflower since school days, we have rediscovered it in a big way. When baked it has a slightly nutty taste, and it makes an ideal replacement for potatoes.

1. Simple roasted cauliflower

Serves 2

1 large cauliflower, broken into florets
1 tbsp olive oil
1 tbsp Parmesan, grated

Preheat the oven to 180°C. Spread the cauliflower over a baking tray, season it with salt and freshly ground black pepper, drizzle over the olive oil and sprinkle with the Parmesan. Roast it for about 20 minutes, turning it halfway through. It is cooked when it has started to soften but is still firm.

- **CALORIES** 130
- PROTEIN 9G
- FAT 8G
- FIBRE 4G
- CARBS 6G

---

2. Spicy roasted cauliflower

Serves 2

2 tbsp coconut, olive or rapeseed oil
Juice of 1 lemon
3 garlic cloves, peeled and halved
1cm root ginger, grated
3 tsp garam masala
1 tsp red chilli, deseeded and finely diced (or 1 tsp chilli flakes)
1 large cauliflower, broken into florets
20g almond flakes

Preheat the oven to 180°C. Mix the oil, lemon juice, garlic and spices together in a good-sized bowl. Add the cauliflower florets, season and mix well together.

Spread the cauliflower over a baking tray and roast it for about 20 minutes, turning it halfway through. It should be al dente. Sprinkle over the almonds 5 minutes before removing the dish from the oven.

Tip: you can add other veg such as broccoli florets or asparagus.

- **CALORIES** 220
- PROTEIN 8G
- FAT 18G
- FIBRE 4G
- CARBS 6G

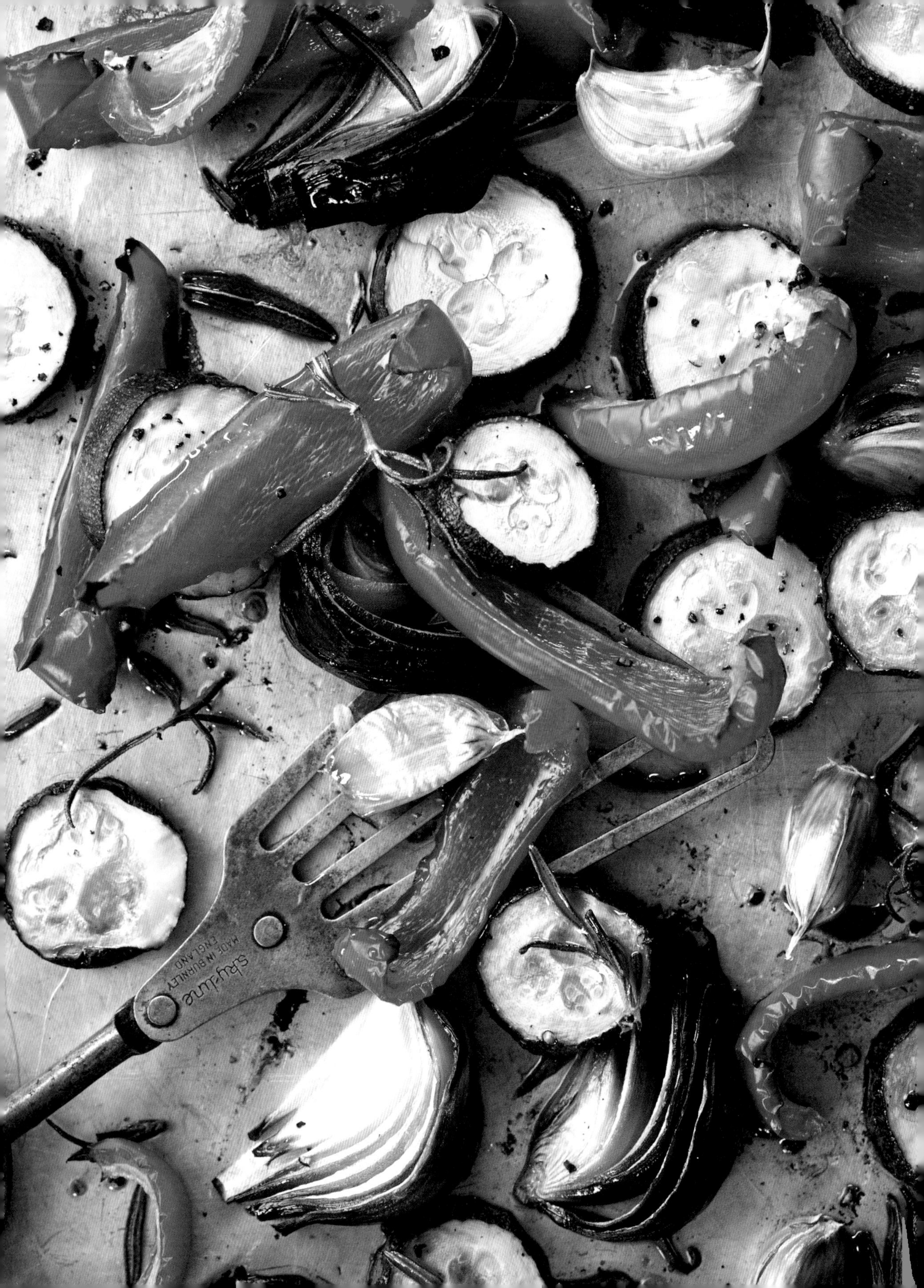
sky-line
MADE IN BURNLEY
ENGLAND

Roasted Mediterranean veg

Serves 4

3 garlic cloves, crushed
3 tbsp olive oil
1 red and 1 yellow pepper, deseeded and quartered
1 aubergine, diced
1 courgette, sliced or diced
1 fennel bulb, sliced
3 tomatoes, quartered
½ red onion, sliced
Sprigs of thyme and rosemary

Preheat the oven to 200°C. In a bowl, mix the garlic with the oil and season with salt and black pepper (and a pinch of chilli flakes if you wish). Arrange the veg in a roasting tin, scatter over the herbs and drizzle with the flavoured oil. Roast for 30-40 minutes, turning once after about 15 minutes.

Tip: when roasting vegetables, make sure you spread them out well on the tray or dish so that they don't go soggy.

- **CALORIES** 130
- PROTEIN 3G
- FAT 9G
- FIBRE 5G
- CARBS 12G

Creamed spinach

Some people find cooked spinach bitter – the crème fraîche counteracts this beautifully.

Serves 2

8 balls of frozen spinach or 200g fresh spinach
Knob of butter or ½ tbsp olive oil
2 heaped tbsp crème fraîche
½ tsp ground nutmeg

If you are using fresh spinach you just need to heat it in a saucepan with the oil or butter for 2-3 minutes, or until it wilts. Defrosting frozen spinach in a saucepan will take a few minutes longer. Drain it well and transfer it to a dish. Stir in the crème fraîche, nutmeg and plenty of seasoning.

Tip: make double quantities as it freezes really well.

- **CALORIES** 160
- PROTEIN 3G
- FAT 15G
- FIBRE 2G
- CARBS 2G

Peas and edamame with yoghurt and lime dressing

Serves 2

50g frozen peas
50g frozen edamame beans
2 tbsp crème fraîche
Handful of dill, chopped
Handful of chives, chopped
Squeeze of lime juice

Put the frozen peas and beans in a pan of boiling water and simmer for 3-4 minutes, then drain them and allow them to cool. In a bowl mix the crème fraîche with the herbs, lime juice and some seasoning, and stir in the peas and beans.

- **CALORIES** 230
- PROTEIN 5G
- FAT 21G
- FIBRE 3G
- CARBS 6G

6 simple ways to get your greens

1. Broccoli with garlic and anchovy

Broccoli contains generous amounts of antioxidant phytochemicals and the more bitter it tastes, the better it is for your health. Unfortunately, to increase sales, most modern supermarket vegetables have had the bitterness bred out of them. This dish is so tasty and nutritious that it could be a meal in itself.

Serves 4

1 tbsp olive oil
1 garlic clove, crushed or chopped
½ tsp red chilli, deseeded and finely diced, or ½ tsp chilli flakes (optional)
2 sprigs of rosemary
3 anchovies from a jar, chopped
200g tenderstem broccoli, long stems included
Squeeze of lemon
1 tbsp pine kernels or flaked almonds, toasted (optional)

In a large pan, heat the oil and sauté the garlic, rosemary and chilli, if using, for a few minutes. Remove the rosemary, add the anchovies and gently simmer for a further 3-5 minutes, crushing the fish into a paste with a wooden spoon as they cook.

Boil, steam or microwave the broccoli for just a couple of minutes, so it retains a slight crunch. Drain it and stir it into the anchovy mixture. Add a generous squeeze of lemon, season and scatter over the toasted nuts or seeds, if using, before serving.

- **CALORIES** 90
- PROTEIN 5G
- FAT 8G
- FIBRE 3G
- CARBS 2G

---

2. Swiss chard stir-fried with garlic

So simple and so good. And it goes with almost anything. Choose fresh seasonal alternatives if possible – kale, spring greens or cabbage also work well.

Serves 2

1 tbsp olive or rapeseed oil
1 garlic clove, crushed or sliced
200g Swiss chard, sliced

Place a frying pan or wok over a high heat, add the oil and fry the garlic for a minute before adding the chard. Turn down the heat to medium, add 1 tbsp warm water and some seasoning and cook it for 2-3 minutes, tossing it frequently, until it is tender but still crisp. Transfer it immediately to a dish and serve.

- **CALORIES** 76
- PROTEIN 3G
- FAT 6G
- FIBRE 2G
- CARBS 2G

3. Cabbage stir-fried Chinese style

Serves 2

1 tbsp coconut or rapeseed oil
1cm root ginger, finely chopped
1 garlic clove, chopped (optional)
½ small cabbage, core removed and leaves finely diced
150g beansprouts
1 tbsp soy sauce
1 tsp sesame oil (optional)

Place a frying pan or wok over a high heat, add the oil and fry the ginger and garlic, if using, for a minute before adding the cabbage. Turn down the heat to medium, add 1 tbsp warm water and cook it for 2 minutes, tossing it frequently, until it is tender but still crisp.

Add the beansprouts and sauté them gently for a minute, before stirring in the soy sauce and sesame oil, if using. Transfer the veg immediately to a dish, season and serve.

- **CALORIES** 80
- PROTEIN 3G
- FAT 6G
- FIBRE 2G
- CARBS 2G

---

4. Pak choi with oyster sauce

This makes an ideal accompaniment to Chinese pork meatballs (see page 85).

Serves 2

1 tbsp coconut or rapeseed oil
200g pak choi or other fresh greens
1 tbsp oyster sauce
1 tsp sesame oil (optional)

Place a frying pan or wok over a high heat, add the oil and then the greens. Turn down the heat to medium, add 1 tbsp warm water and cook for 2 minutes, tossing them frequently. Then stir in the oyster sauce and drizzle over the sesame oil, if using. The greens are done when they are tender but still crisp. Transfer them to a dish and serve immediately.

- **CALORIES** 170
- PROTEIN 4G
- FAT 12G
- FIBRE 5G
- CARBS 11G

5. Spring greens with garlic and cannellini beans

Beans make up an important part of the Mediterranean-style diet and work really well slipped into a dish to add taste and texture. They also make it significantly more filling.

Serves 2

1 tbsp olive oil
1 garlic clove, crushed
½ tsp chilli flakes
½ tsp dried thyme or oregano
8 cherry tomatoes, halved
100g cannellini beans (just under ½ tin, rinsed and drained)
200g spring greens, finely sliced, or mature spinach
Squeeze of lemon

Heat the oil in a saucepan with a lid and add the garlic, chilli flakes and thyme or oregano, followed by the tomatoes, beans and greens. Then add ½ tbsp water and a generous squeeze of lemon and some seasoning.

Stir and simmer gently with the lid on until the greens are cooked (around 2-3 minutes) or just wilted. Transfer them to a dish and serve.

- **CALORIES** 130
- PROTEIN 7G
- FAT 7G
- FIBRE 6G
- CARBS 12G

---

6. Green beans with soy sauce and sesame seeds

An adaptation of a lovely Japanese recipe given to us by chef Akemi Yokoyama. Delicious, quick and easy.

Serves 2

200g thin French beans, cut in half, or mange tout
2 tbsp white sesame seeds
1 tbsp soy sauce
1 tsp sesame oil
1 tsp hoisin plum sauce (or ½ tsp maple syrup)

Bring a pan of water to the boil and add the beans with a pinch of salt. Cook them for 3 minutes (less for mange tout) over a medium heat or until they are just tender. Then run them under cold water in a sieve, drain them and leave them to one side.

Dry-roast the sesame seeds in a frying pan or wok over a low heat, stirring all the time. Remove them as soon as they start to brown (after about 1 minute) and immediately transfer them to a dish to stop them from burning.

Using the same pan, turn up the heat to medium and throw in the beans with the sesame oil, then add the soy sauce and plum sauce. Sauté for 1 minute, and season to taste. Serve immediately.

- **CALORIES** 120
- PROTEIN 6G
- FAT 9G
- FIBRE 3G
- CARBS 6G

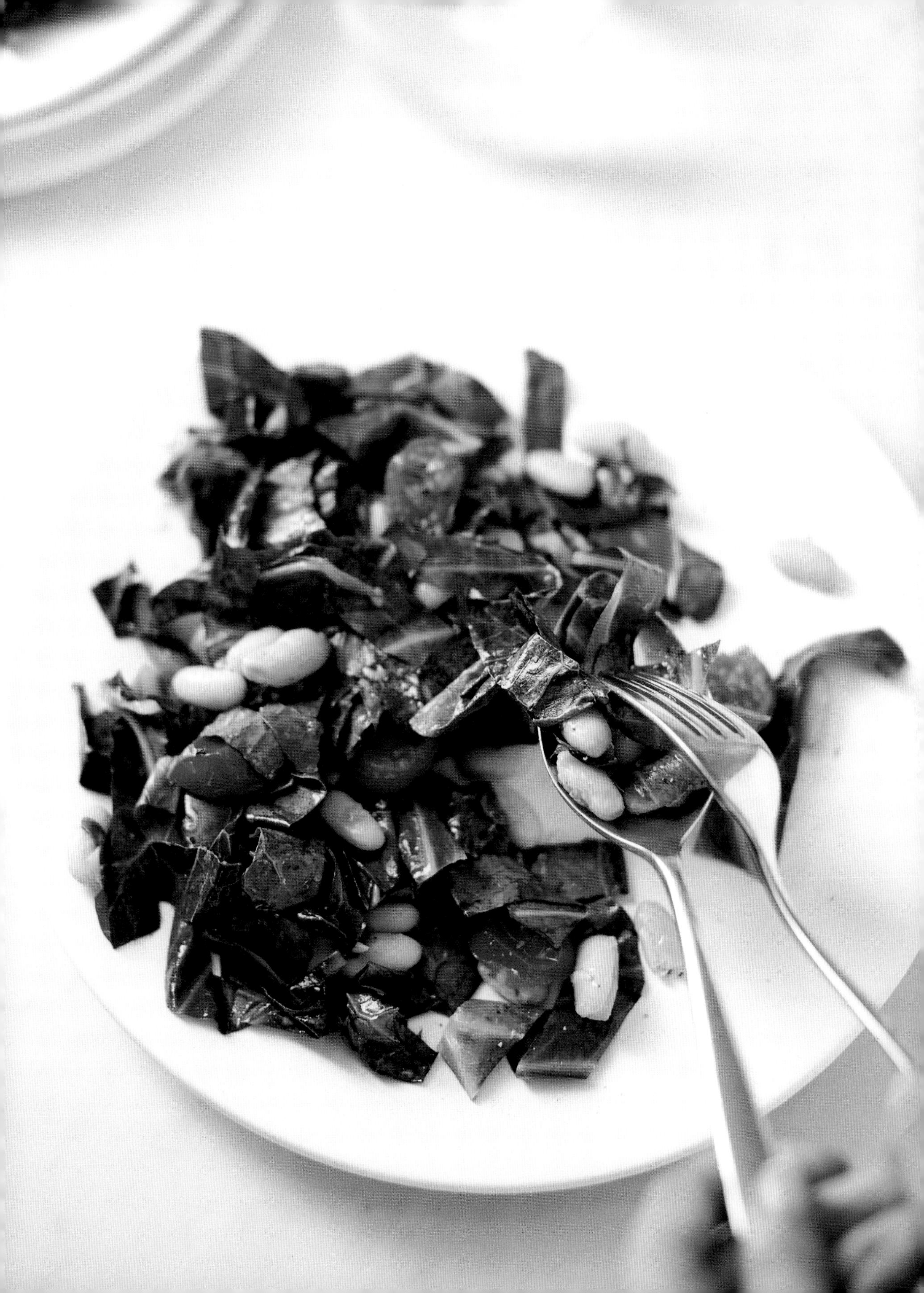

Dressings

Some dressings require a small amount of sugar or honey to counteract the vinegar or lemon. Although this goes somewhat against the principles of the Blood Sugar Diet, if it helps you enjoy and eat more vegetables then it is a compromise worth making. In the scheme of things half a teaspoon of maple syrup or honey in a dressing is insignificant, as part of a meal.

Mayo 4 ways

It's wonderful to have mayonnaise back on the menu, now that we are being encouraged to eat more healthy fats with our food. You can of course make your own, but a good-quality shop-bought mayo works well, particularly if you add different flavours to it. Remember that full-fat is better for you and tastes better too, though it is also high in calories so watch the quantities.

All the following make 2 portions

1. Light lemon mayo

Perfect with asparagus tips.

Zest of 1 lemon
1 tbsp full-fat mayonnaise
1 tbsp full-fat Greek yoghurt

Beat all the ingredients together and adjust the seasoning.

- **CALORIES** 75
- PROTEIN 2G
- FAT 8G
- FIBRE 0G
- CARBS 1G

2. Garlic mayo

2 tbsp full-fat mayonnaise
1 tbsp full-fat Greek yoghurt
½ garlic clove, crushed
1 tbsp chives or dill, chopped (optional)

Beat all the ingredients together and adjust the seasoning.

- **CALORIES** 130
- PROTEIN 1G
- FAT 14G
- FIBRE 0G
- CARBS 1G

3. Anchovy mayo

1 tbsp full-fat mayonnaise
1 tbsp olive oil
1 tbsp lime or lemon juice
6 anchovies from a jar or tin, finely chopped
1 level tbsp rosemary leaves, very finely chopped

Mix together the mayo, oil and lime or lemon juice to form a creamy texture, add the rest of the ingredients with some freshly ground black pepper and mix together energetically to infuse the flavours.

- **CALORIES 150**
- PROTEIN 2G
- FAT 16
- FIBRE 0G
- CARBS 0G

4. Chilli mayo

Great as a dip or with seafood. Worth making the sweet chilli sauce for this alone.

1 tbsp low-sugar sweet chilli sauce (see page 175)
1 tbsp full-fat mayonnaise

Beat all the ingredients together and adjust the seasoning.

- **CALORIES** 105
- PROTEIN 1G
- FAT 10G
- FIBRE 0G
- CARBS 1G

French vinaigrette

Makes 4 portions

4 tbsp olive oil
2 tbsp lemon juice
1 tsp English, Dijon or wholegrain mustard
¼ garlic clove, crushed (optional)

Beat all the ingredients together and adjust the seasoning.

- **CALORIES** 100
- PROTEIN 0G
- FAT 11G
- FIBRE 0G
- CARBS 2G

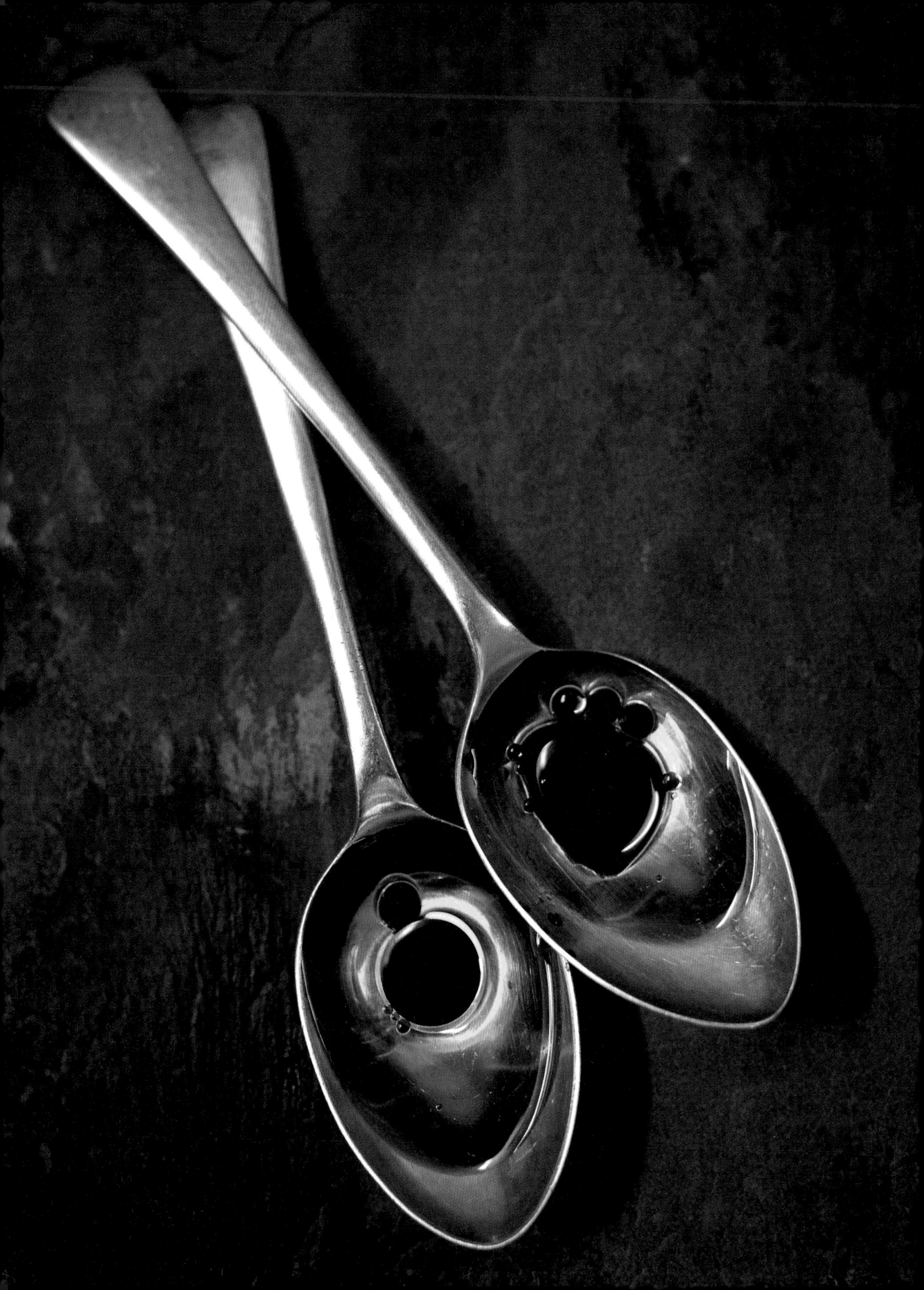

Yoghurt 2 ways

Makes 2 portions

1. Yoghurt and mustard dressing

2 tsp English mustard
½ tbsp olive oil
½ tbsp walnut oil
1 tbsp full-fat natural yoghurt

- CALORIES 70
- PROTEIN 1G
- FAT 3G
- FIBRE 0G
- CARBS 1G

2. Garlic and lemon yoghurt dressing

2 tbsp full-fat Greek yoghurt
½ garlic clove, crushed
Zest of half a lemon
1 mint leaf, finely chopped (optional)

- CALORIES 40
- PROTEIN 2G
- FAT 3G
- FIBRE 0G
- CARBS 1G

Low-sugar sweet chilli sauce

Makes 6 portions

Instead of cornflour, this recipe uses the natural thickening properties of chia seeds, so it contains very little starchy carbohydrate. It tastes as good, is easier to make and remarkably authentic.

1-2 red chillies, deseeded and very finely diced
½ small red pepper, deseeded and very finely diced
1cm root ginger, grated
1 garlic clove, crushed
1 tsp chia seeds
1 tbsp balsamic vinegar
1 tbsp mirin wine
¼ tsp salt
1 tbsp Thai fish sauce

Place all the ingredients in a pan along with 2 tbsp water, cover and simmer gently for 4-5 minutes, stirring regularly (or microwave for 3-4 minutes). Add an extra tbsp water gradually if the consistency is too thick. Pour the sauce into a clean glass container with a lid and store it in the fridge.

Tip: chia seeds have an extraordinary ability to absorb fluid to form a gel, ideal for thickening a sauce. If you don't have any, stir in 1 tsp cornflour instead.

- CALORIES 40
- PROTEIN 1G
- FAT 2G
- FIBRE 2G
- CARBS 1G

Buttermilk dressing

The live cultured buttermilk gives this dressing a wonderful creamy tangy taste. Fermented milk not only improves our ability to absorb nutrients but also helps restore the balance of healthy bacteria in our gut. What's more, it contains significantly fewer calories than whole milk.

Makes 4 portions

60ml buttermilk
50g full-fat mayonnaise
1 tbsp cider vinegar
½ tsp maple syrup (optional)

Mix all the ingredients together with a generous pinch of salt and black pepper.

- **CALORIES** 70
- PROTEIN 1G
- FAT 6G
- FIBRE 0G
- CARBS 1G

Red salsa

So much nicer than the shop-bought version.

Makes 2 portions

150g tomatoes, finely chopped
½ garlic clove, chopped
½ tbsp cider vinegar
2 tbsp olive oil
½ small red pepper, deseeded and diced
½ tsp red chilli, deseeded and finely diced (or ½ tsp chilli flakes), to taste
Handful of parsley or coriander, chopped

Mix all the ingredients together in a bowl and season with salt and black pepper.

- **CALORIES** 140
- PROTEIN 1G
- FAT 13G
- FIBRE 2G
- CARBS 5G

Home-made pesto

Easy to make and bursting with flavour.

Makes 4 portions

50g chopped walnuts, toasted
50g pine nuts, toasted
50g basil leaves, chopped
5 tbsp olive oil
Juice of 2 lemons

Blitz all the ingredients with a hand blender or in a food processor. Season, and store in a clean jar in the fridge for a few days or in the freezer.

- CALORIES 160
- PROTEIN 2G
- FAT 17G
- FIBRE 0G
- CARBS 1G

Toppings

Scatter these on top of soups, fish, vegetables or salads to add extra flavour.

- **Chorizo or black pudding:** great with white fish or scallops, or on top of soups. 20g chorizo or black pudding, very finely chopped and roasted or fried (= 60 cals)
- **Pancetta:** these add flavour and extra protein to soup, and are delicious scattered on a bake or salad. 20g pancetta fried gently in a dash of olive oil until crispy and golden brown, with a crushed garlic clove for extra flavour (= 70 cals)
- **Roasted nuts and seeds:** the toasting brings out the flavours, giving them a sweet and nutty taste. Keep them in an airtight jam jar. Half a handful of sesame seeds, pine nuts, pumpkin, chia or other seeds (either grilled on a tray or baked in the oven, or dry-roasted in a non-stick frying pan).
- **Diced feta** (30g = 80 cals) or **fried halloumi cheese** (40g = 130 cals)
- **Garlic-sautéed kale:** to sprinkle on top of soups. 50g kale, leaves torn off and sautéed for a few minutes in 1 tsp olive oil with a crushed garlic clove (= 50 cals)
- **Sliced mushrooms:** 50g finely sliced mushrooms sautéed in a dollop of butter with a chopped garlic clove, garnished with finely chopped parsley (= 50 calories)

Occasional Treats

This chapter is all about showing you that, even while on the Blood Sugar Diet, you can eat occasional treats, our thinking being that it is better to have the odd cake or pudding which is low in sugar and relatively low-carb than risk being tempted by sweet, carb-rich alternatives.

Bread is more tricky, because it is an everyday food that people generally find it much harder to cut down on. The more you train yourself to do without it, the better your chances of keeping the weight off in the long term. So we recommend that while you are on the 800-calorie-a-day regime you keep your bread intake to an absolute minimum. If and when you do eat bread, make it the relatively solid and chewy kind containing unrefined wholegrains and seeds, like those we have included here.

Roasted rhubarb with ginger, see page 194

Breads and flatbread

There are now so many different flours available – not just wheat and rye, but also nut varieties, such as coconut, almond or chestnut – that making a choice can be daunting. The flours come in different degrees of 'refinement', from coarsely chopped, to ground, to fully refined. This affects how much fibre remains in them and whether the healthy oils and nutrients have been removed or not. The amount of processing will also determine whether they are low or high GI and how great a sugar spike they cause.

If you are used to standard processed wheat flour you will find that nut flours behave differently when used for baking. Some absorb lots of fluid, some have a grainy texture and, to make things even more complicated, the proportions of flour to liquid required are often not quite equivalent. Stick closely to the recipes, and you will be fine!

Wholegrain soda bread

According to Elizabeth David, 'Everyone who cooks should know how to make a loaf of soda bread.' It really is easy. It doesn't require yeast, or kneading or time to rise.

Makes 12 slices
(cals are per slice)

325g wholemeal flour
75g wholemeal spelt flour
2 tbsp rolled oats
2 tsp bicarbonate of soda
½ tsp salt
2 tbsp pumpkin seeds, plus extra for sprinkling
2 tbsp sunflower seeds, plus extra for sprinkling
75g walnuts, chopped
325ml buttermilk
3-4 tbsp milk
1 tbsp olive oil

Preheat the oven to 230°C. Place the flours, oats, bicarbonate of soda and salt in a mixing bowl with the seeds and walnuts. Stir in the buttermilk. Mix gently to make a soft dough, adding the milk gradually. Shape the dough on a floured surface and place it in an oiled 900g loaf tin. Alternatively, shape it into a flattened ball and cut a cross into the surface for a more traditional shape. Scatter the rest of the seeds over the work surface and roll the loaf over them so they stick to it.

Bake the loaf in the oven for 10 minutes, then reduce the temperature to 200°C and bake it for a further 20-30 minutes, until it is golden and firm.

Tip: we suggest you slice any bread you don't eat and keep it in a bag in the freezer. Cooling the bread will also convert some of the starchy carbohydrate in it into more fibrous 'resistant starch' which has less impact on blood sugar (note – only some of the starch!).

- **CALORIES** 210
- PROTEIN 7G
- FAT 8G
- FIBRE 3G
- CARBS 29G

Seeded spelt and rye bread

Spelt or hulled wheat, cultivated since 5000 BC, is a hardier and more nutritious cousin of modern wheat and has a sweetish, slightly nutty taste. This bread, adapted from a lovely recipe by JPS Cloud on the website, is easy to make, particularly in a breadmaker. You can adjust the proportions of the flour – just note that the more rye you add, the less it rises.

Makes 12 slices
(cals are per slice)

400g stoneground spelt flour
120g stoneground rye flour
1½ tsp salt
2 tsp yeast
3 tbsp seeds of your choice: we suggest 1 tbsp poppy (these are small and don't overwhelm the bread), 1 tbsp sunflower and 1 tbsp linseeds or pumpkin
430ml lukewarm water
2 tbsp olive oil (or 40g butter)
1 tbsp honey

Put all the ingredients in the breadmaker tin and set as a 'large' loaf on the wholemeal cycle (takes 4-5 hours, depending on the breadmaker). Easy.

Or you can bake it in the oven. Put the flour, salt, seeds and yeast in a large bowl and mix them together. Then gradually stir in the lukewarm water along with the oil and the honey to form a dough. Use your hands to finish mixing it. There should be none left sticking to the bowl.

Transfer the dough to a flat surface scattered lightly with flour and knead it for 5 minutes, until it no longer feels sticky. Add more flour as needed. Oil the loaf tin and fold the dough into a shape that fits inside it, pressing it in evenly. Put it in a large plastic food bag and leave it to rise for 2 hours (until the dough no longer springs back when you press it with your finger). Then remove it from the bag and place it in an oven preheated to 200°C.

Remove the tin after about 35-40 minutes. It should have risen and turned golden brown. Tip the bread out onto the baking tray. It should sound hollow when you tap it. If you like crisp crusts, put it back in the oven for 5 more minutes.

Tip: kneading bread should be a bit of an upper body workout as you need to repeatedly stretch the dough by pushing it away from you with the base of your hand, then fold it onto itself and repeat, for at least 5 minutes.

- **CALORIES** 180
- PROTEIN 5G
- FAT 5G
- FIBRE 4G
- CARBS 30G

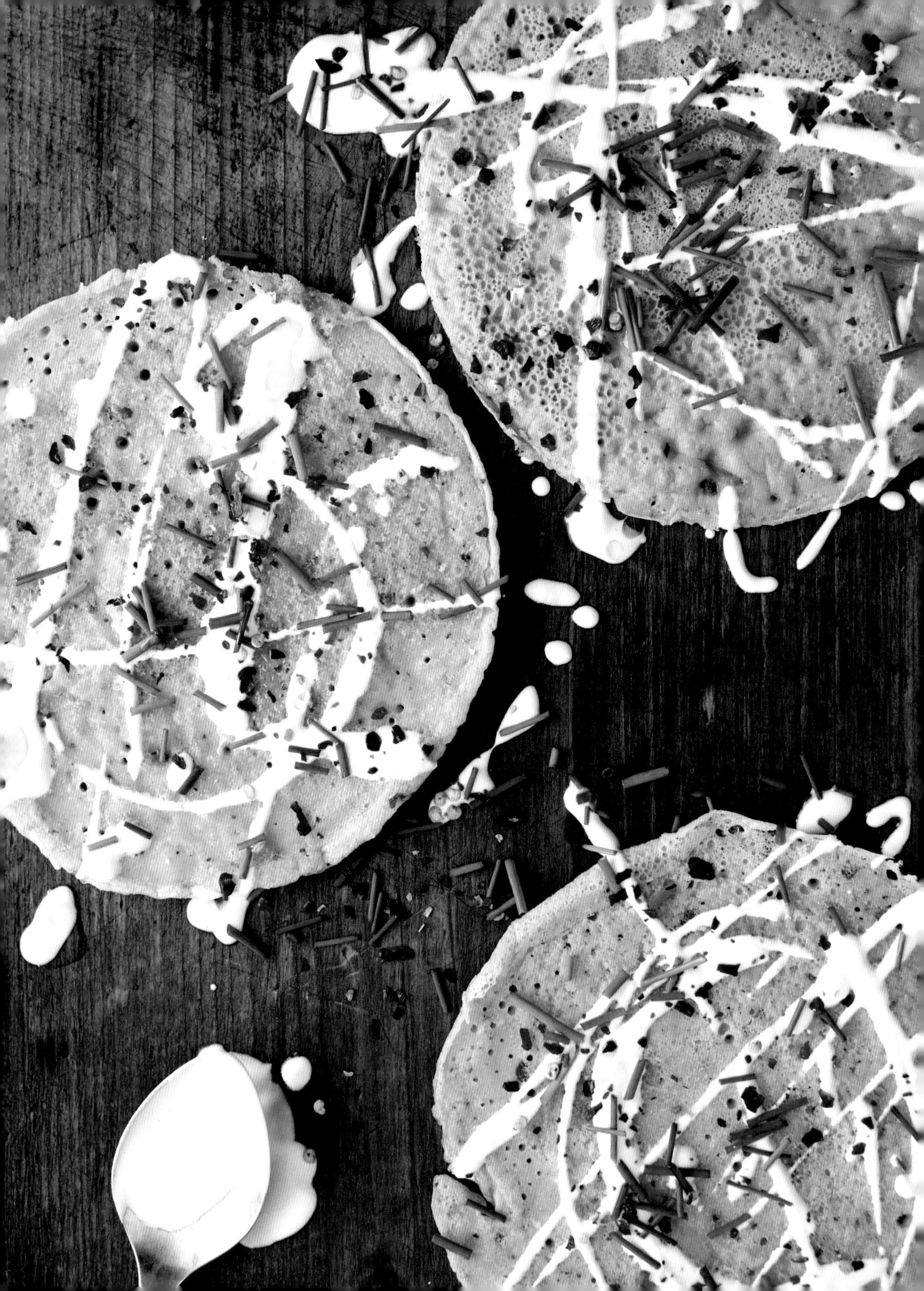

Chickpea flatbread

Many of my Asian patients with blood sugar problems tell me that they struggle to replace flatbreads or chapattis in their diet. Unfortunately, most shop-bought flatbreads these days are made of highly refined wheat flour, whereas in India they are traditionally made with wholemeal chickpea flour, which is relatively lower in carbohydrate and high in protein and fibre. It is also gluten-free. This is what we have used here. Chickpea flour can be found online and in most health food shops and Asian supermarkets. This is adapted from an excellent recipe posted online by Ingenue.

Makes 8

250g chickpea flour (also known as gram flour or besan)
Water (enough to make a thin batter)
Pinch of salt
Seasoning: we use pinches of chilli flakes, pepper and onion powder, and either rosemary or caraway seeds.
1 tbsp coconut or olive oil

Put the chickpea flour in a bowl and add enough water to make a thin pancake batter, whisking well as you go. Add the salt and seasoning, and then leave it to stand for 2-3 hours. When you are ready to use it, whisk in the oil. Put a frying pan on a medium-high heat. If the pan is not non-stick, lightly brush it with olive oil. Swirl the batter into the pan and cook it until it is brown and crisp, turning once.

Tip: these can also be used as pizza bases, or as wraps to fill with salad, tuna and mayonnaise or other healthy choices. They freeze well.

- **CALORIES** 110
- PROTEIN 6G
- FAT 3G
- FIBRE 3G
- CARBS 16G

Puddings for now and then

Eat them slowly, in small portions – and enjoy!

Instant creamy passion fruit pudding

Incredibly easy to assemble – and looks very inviting layered in a glass.

Serves 1

2 tbsp crème fraîche (or full-fat coconut yoghurt)
1 passion fruit
Handful of berries
½ mint leaf, finely chopped
½ tsp maple syrup (optional and ideally skipped!)

Put the crème fraîche in a small glass. Cut the passion fruit in half, scoop out the seeds and juice and tip them onto the crème fraîche. Scatter the berries and the mint on top and drizzle over the maple syrup, if using.

- CALORIES 240
- PROTEIN 2G
- FAT 24G
- FIBRE 1G
- CARBS 5G

Quick chia kulfi

Inspired by a pistachio kulfi, a delightful dessert that we ate at an Indian restaurant recently. This is an easy alternative, with a similarly delicate exotic flavour and no added sugar.

Serves 2

160ml tin coconut cream
20g pistachios (15g of these crushed)
1½ tsp chia seeds
Seeds from 3 cardamom pods
Pinch of salt
Small handful of berries (optional)

In a small pan gently heat the coconut milk, crushed pistachios, chia and cardamom seeds. Add the salt and simmer for about 5 minutes. Pour the mixture into 2 small bowls or ramekins and place them in the fridge for 1-2 hours to set. Scatter the remaining pistachios and the berries, if using, over the top.

Tip: to deseed the cardamom, crush the pod gently with the flat of a knife, then tip out the seeds.

- CALORIES 360
- PROTEIN 6G
- FAT 36G
- FIBRE 1G
- CARBS 6G

Orange and pistachio cupcakes

These have an exotic taste, reminiscent of a North African sweet treat, but without the syrup. They are very low-carb and contain a satisfying amount of protein.

Makes 6
(calories are per cake)

1 large or 2 small eggs
2 tbsp coconut oil (or butter, melted)
Zest and juice of 1 orange
5 large pitted dates, very finely chopped
100g ground almonds
1 tsp baking powder
Seeds from 3 cardamom pods
25g pistachios, roughly crushed
6 good-sized raspberries
¼ tsp salt

Preheat the oven to 170°C. Mix all the moist ingredients with the dates and blitz them with a hand blender or in a food processor (or with a fork). Then stir in the dry ingredients along with half of the pistachios. Mix everything together vigorously. Spoon the mixture into 6 cupcake cases and set them aside for a few minutes to let the baking powder act. Press a raspberry into the middle of each cupcake and scatter the remaining pistachios on top. Bake the cakes for about 15 minutes. They are done when they are golden brown and springy to the touch.

- **CALORIES** 360
- PROTEIN 10G
- FAT 25G
- FIBRE 4G
- CARBS 25G

Almond pancakes with cherries

Serves 4

50g cherries, halved and stones removed
2 eggs
250ml almond milk (or dairy milk)
1 tbsp vanilla extract
100g almond flour
Pinch of baking powder
Coconut oil or butter for frying
2 tbsp fromage frais

Put the cherries in a small saucepan with a splash of water and gently simmer to make a soft jam. Whisk the eggs, almond milk and vanilla extract together in a bowl. Then add the almond flour and baking powder and combine well to make a smooth batter.

Place a large non-stick frying pan over a medium heat and add a little coconut oil or butter, tipping the pan so that it is evenly coated. When it starts to smoke, add a ladle of the batter, again tipping the pan to spread it over the entire surface. After about a minute, when the underside is golden brown, flip it over and cook the other side for another minute. Serve with the cherries and fromage frais.

Tip: you can use berries instead of cherries or use the berry coulis on page 189.

- **CALORIES** 170
- PROTEIN 6G
- FAT 7G
- FIBRE 0G
- CARBS 40G

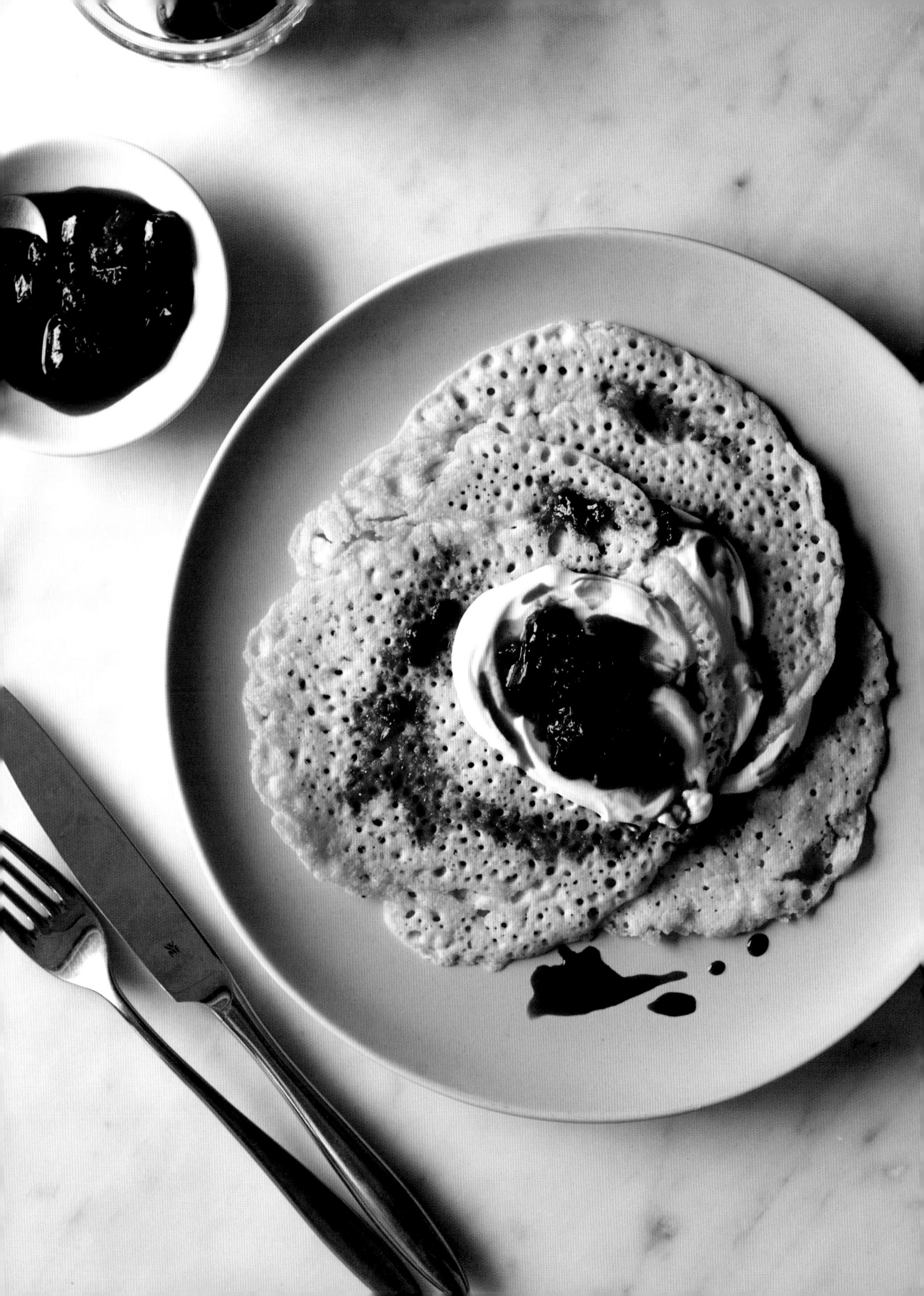

Pumpkin pudding with crunchy nut topping

Inspired by the American classic, this is still full of autumnal flavour, but won't send your blood sugars soaring.

Serves 8

½ small pumpkin (500g), peeled and diced
100g or 12 soft dried apricots, quartered
3 large eggs
200ml coconut milk
Juice of half a lemon (and zest, optional)
2 tsp mixed spice
25g pumpkin seeds
25g pecans, chopped
2 tsp maple syrup (optional)
Pinch of salt

Preheat the oven to 180°C. Place the pumpkin on a baking tray, add a splash of water and cover it with foil. Make a small steam hole in the middle of the foil and bake the pumpkin for 45 minutes. Put it aside to cool. Meanwhile, soak the apricots in hot water for 5-10 minutes.

Blend the cooled pumpkin with the apricots, eggs, coconut milk, lemon and mixed spice in a food processor. Pour the mixture into 8 ramekins and place them on an oven tray. Pour boiling water into the tray until it comes halfway up the side of the ramekins. Bake them in the oven for 30 minutes, then carefully remove the tray from the oven and place the ramekins in the fridge for 3-4 hours to completely chill.

Put the pumpkin seeds and pecans in a small ovenproof dish and toss them in the maple syrup, if using. Roast them in the oven for about 15 minutes, or until they turn golden brown. Scatter them on top of the puddings before serving.

Tips: this pudding can also be made with butternut squash, which is available all year round, but try and make the most of pumpkin when it's in season. Baking is better than boiling as it caramelises the pumpkin/squash and makes it taste sweeter. For convenience you can now buy bags of ready-diced butternut squash.

- **CALORIES** 140
- PROTEIN 4G
- FAT 10G
- FIBRE 2G
- CARBS 8G

Berry coulis or 'jam'

A peculiar property of chia is its ability to expand and absorb fluid, forming a clear gel. As it has no particular taste, it takes on the flavours of the other ingredients. So here we use it to make a berry coulis, as a delicious alternative to jam to drizzle into yoghurt or over a pudding. It's quick to make and requires no cornflour or starch for thickening.

Serves 4

100g berries with seeds (frozen is fine)
1 tsp chia seeds for a coulis, 2 tsp for 'jam'
50ml water
½-1 tsp maple syrup (optional)

Put the berries and water in a small pan and bring to the boil. When the berries begin to soften, mash them with a fork or potato masher, then add the chia seeds. Simmer the mixture for about 5 minutes, adding more water if it gets too thick. You can add maple syrup for a touch of sweetness if you feel you need to. The coulis/jam can be stored in a jar in the fridge for a few days.

Tip: make a berry 'mousse' by stirring half of one serving of berry coulis into 2 tbsp crème fraîche, then drizzling the other half on top. Easy.

- **CALORIES** 20
- PROTEIN 1G
- FAT 1G
- FIBRE 1G
- CARBS 3G

Chocolate kidney bean cake

We cooked this for a bunch of teenagers who liked it and never got close to guessing that the main ingredient was kidney beans.

Serves 12

400g tin red kidney beans, drained and rinsed
1 tbsp vanilla extract
5 eggs
150g coconut oil
15 soft pitted dates, diced
60g cocoa powder
1 tsp baking powder
½ tsp ground cinnamon
Pinch of salt
150g fresh raspberries or cherries, stones removed

Preheat the oven to 150°C. Grease a 20cm round cake tin and line the base with lightly greased greaseproof paper. In a moderate-sized bowl blend the kidney beans, vanilla extract, 2 eggs, 1 tbsp water and the coconut oil until smooth (about 4-5 minutes). Then add the rest of the ingredients and mix them together well.

Pour the mixture into the cake tin, gently press the raspberries into the surface then bake it for about 30 minutes. Remove the cake from the oven and leave it to cool for 10 minutes before turning it out on a rack.

Tip: you can also use this mixture to make cupcakes. Use a 12-hole tray, lined with paper cases. They need slightly less cooking time: 15-20 mins.

- **CALORIES** 250
- PROTEIN 7G
- FAT 16G
- FIBRE 4G
- CARBS 20G

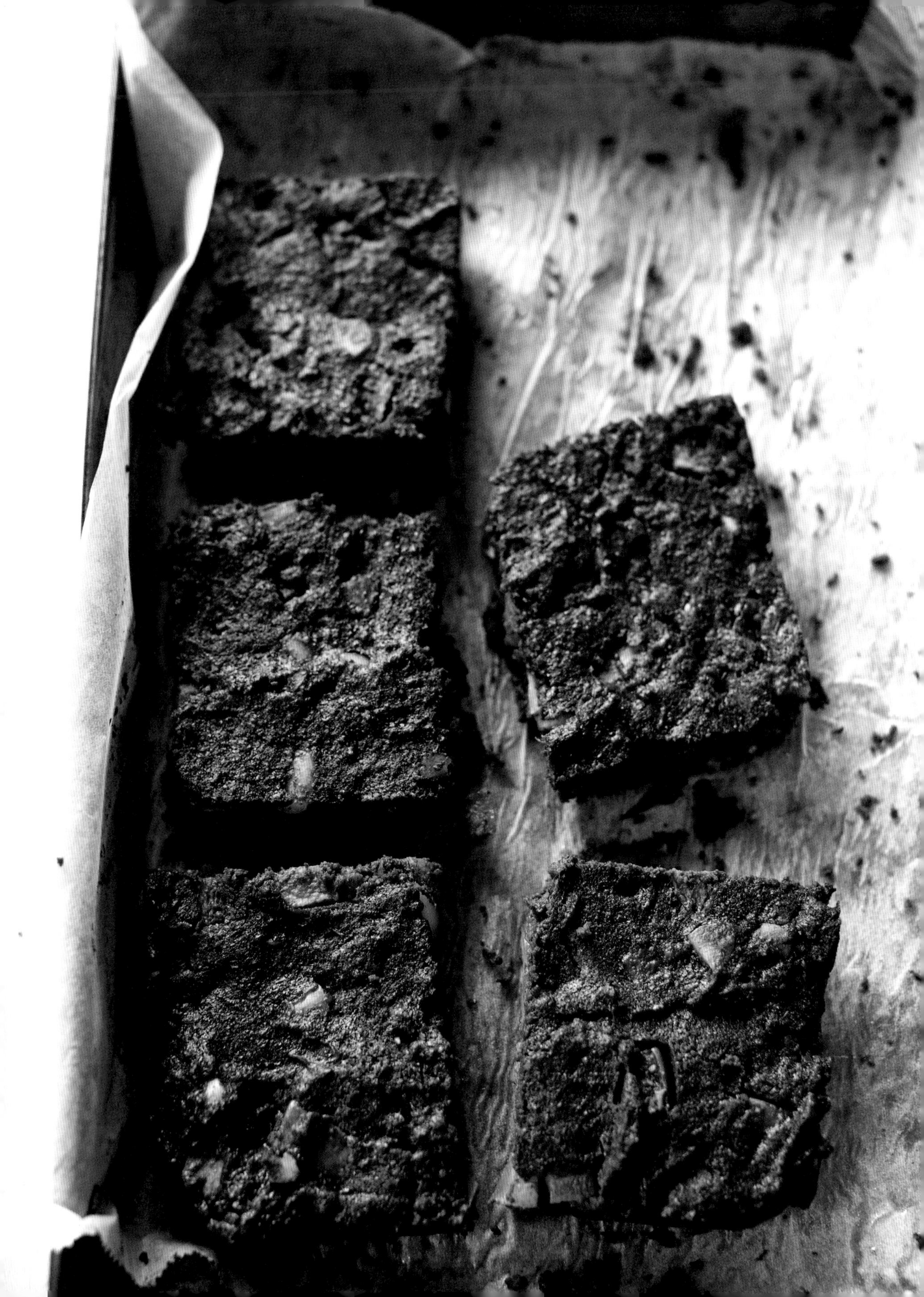

Pear and Brazil nut chocolate brownies

The pear and Brazil nuts give these brownies a lovely subtle flavour. And what's more, Brazil nuts are an excellent source of minerals, particularly selenium (important for thyroid function and the immune system). Cut the brownies small and freeze any left over. They make a great after-dinner treat.

Makes 16
(calories per brownie)

60g pitted dates, finely chopped
60g coconut oil (or unsalted butter, softened), plus extra to grease
3 eggs
100g ground almonds
1 pear, quartered and cored, skin on
140g dark chocolate (70% cocoa solids)
25g Brazil nuts, chopped
Pinch of salt

Preheat the oven to 180°C and grease a 20cm square cake tin. Put the dates in a small saucepan with a splash of water. Cover and gently simmer for 3-5 minutes or until they soften. Allow them to cool, then blend them with the coconut oil in a food processor or with a hand blender. Transfer the mixture to a large bowl and add the eggs, then the ground almonds, and beat until everything is incorporated. Dice the pear into ½cm squares and stir it into the mixture too, along with the Brazil nuts.

Melt the dark chocolate in a heatproof bowl set over, but not touching, a pan of steaming water (or microwave it on a medium heat for 1-2 minutes). Allow it to cool a bit before stirring it into the brownie mixture. Pour the mixture into the tin and bake it for 15-20 minutes, or until a knife comes out clean. Delicious with a dollop of crème fraîche (adds 90 calories).

- **CALORIES** 155
- PROTEIN 3G
- FAT 12G
- FIBRE 1G
- CARBS 10G

A word on fruit and sugar…

For some reason fruit always comes first in the 'eat more fruit and veg' recommendations. In our view, this is the wrong way round. Unfortunately, some people are eating huge amounts of fruit, believing that it's doing them good. I have seen patients whose blood sugars return to normal simply by cutting right down on their fruit consumption.

Fruit contains lots of beneficial nutrients, but you can almost certainly get these from eating just 1-2 portions a day. Try and stick to the lower-sugar fruits, such as berries, grapes and pears. When you are looking to add flavour or sweetness to a dish, we recommend you go for fruits such as cranberries, prunes, dates, pomegranates, goji berries, raisins and occasionally, if there is no alternative, a teaspoon of maple syrup or honey.

As you reduce your sugar intake, you will find you start to enjoy different flavours in your food and that you can reduce the tart or bitter taste of some fruit by adding dairy products or the soya or coconut equivalents, which act as a natural sweetener.

We would suggest that you avoid artificial sweeteners entirely. One of the main problems with them is that they are so many times sweeter than normal sugar that they maintain sugar cravings. Ideally, also avoid syrups such as agave or concentrated fruit juice, as these tend to have a very high GI.

When in doubt, go for the whole unprocessed fruit, which is released far more slowly and contains more fibre so has less impact on blood sugars, especially if eaten as part of a meal.

Lychee and pink grapefruit salad

A light exotic-tasting fruit salad which can be assembled in just a few minutes from items you can pull out of the cupboard. Some research suggests that grapefruit helps lower cholesterol.*

Serves 4

400g tin lychees, drained
400g tin grapefruit in fruit juice, not syrup (pink grapefruit works best)
Seeds from 2 cardamom pods
½-1 tsp lime zest, ideally in fine strips

Put the grapefruit and its juice in a bowl along with the lychees (without their juice) and the cardamom seeds. To make the lime strips, dig the top edge of a potato peeler into the surface of the lime at an angle and scrape off a fine thread or twist of zest. It looks lovely strewn among the fruit. Alternatively, use a smaller quantity of finely grated zest. If time allows, cover the fruit and leave the flavours to merge for about 30 minutes.

Tip: tinned lychees are not always available in the supermarket so grab a few tins when you see them (fresh are delicious if you can find them, but fiddly to peel).

- **CALORIES** 100
- PROTEIN 1G
- FAT 0G
- FIBRE 1G
- CARBS 25G

Fruit sponge pudding

We cook this at home a lot as it can be made with frozen fruit such as plums, rhubarb and blackberries. The sponge is made with ground almonds which is the least processed of the almond flours and retains more of its healthy oils and fibre. It has a delicious flavour and a slightly chewy texture, which works well with the baked fruit.

Serves 6

400g plums, halved and stoned
100g coconut oil (or butter)
2 eggs
Zest of 1 lemon
100g pitted dates, finely chopped
100g ground almonds
1 tsp ground cinnamon (optional)
1 tsp baking powder

Preheat the oven to 160°C. Place the fruit in a greased 20cm ovenproof dish. Beat together the coconut oil or butter, eggs and lemon zest. Stir in the dates, ground almonds, cinnamon, if using, and baking powder and mix well. Spoon the mixture on top of the fruit. Bake the pudding for 35-40 minutes. Serve it with 1 tbsp full-fat Greek yoghurt (adds 30 calories) or crème fraîche (adds 90 calories).

Tips: frozen fruit is just as healthy and can be more convenient if it is ready chopped. Cinnamon is thought to help reduce blood sugars.

- **CALORIES** 350
- PROTEIN 7G
- FAT 28G
- FIBRE 3G
- CARBS 18G

---

* However, it can interact with certain medications. Please consult your doctor if you are at risk.

Roasted fruit

Roasted peaches (or apricots)

Serves 4

1 tbsp coconut oil (or butter), plus extra for greasing
Handful of pistachios, roughly crushed or chopped
4 pitted dates, finely chopped
4 ripe peaches or 6 ripe apricots, halved and stones removed

Preheat the oven to 180°C. Grease a baking dish with coconut oil or butter. Mix the coconut oil, nuts and dates together in a bowl. Place the fruit halves in the baking dish cut side up and fill the stone cavities with the date and nut mixture. Pour 100ml water around the fruit and bake it for 20-30 minutes or until it starts to brown. Serve with 1 tbsp crème fraîche (adds 90 calories) or Greek yoghurt (adds 30 calories).

- **CALORIES** 90
- PROTEIN 2G
- FAT 6G
- FIBRE 2G
- CARBS 9G

Roasted rhubarb with ginger

This is so good you might be tempted to lick the dish. The rhubarb and ginger caramelise and char slightly, and are perfect served with a dollop of crème fraîche.

Serves 2

200g rhubarb, cut at an angle into 3cm pieces
1 tbsp coconut oil (or butter, melted)
Knob of ginger in syrup, drained

Preheat the oven to 180°C. Spread the rhubarb on a baking tray and pour the coconut oil over it. Slice the ginger into fine matchsticks and scatter it over the rhubarb. Bake the rhubarb for 20-30 minutes and serve it with 1 tbsp crème fraîche (adds 90 calories) or Greek yoghurt (adds 30 calories).

- **CALORIES** 50
- PROTEIN 2G
- FAT 4G
- FIBRE 2G
- CARBS 5G

Baked spiced apple with nuts

Serves 2

2 medium cooking apples
4 Medjool dates, pitted and chopped
1 tbsp ground almonds
1 tsp ground cinnamon
½ tsp freshly ground nutmeg (if you have it)
20g pecans or walnuts, chopped
1 tsp vanilla extract

Preheat the oven to 160°C. Core the apples, making the hole about 2cm in diameter, so there is enough room for the stuffing, and put them in a baking dish. Place the dates in a small saucepan with 1 tbsp of water and gently simmer them to form a purée. Stir in the rest of the ingredients, then fill the apples with the mixture. Bake the apples, uncovered, for approximately 40-50 minutes. If a knife slides through the flesh fairly easily, they are done. Serve with 1 tbsp Greek yoghurt (adds 30 calories), or the coconut or soya equivalent.

- **CALORIES** 260
- PROTEIN 4G
- FAT 13G
- FIBRE 4G
- CARBS 33G

Swaps and tips

Carb alternatives

Below is a list of our favourite alternatives to pasta, rice, noodles and potatoes, some of which you will already have encountered in earlier chapters.

Cauliflower mash

Serves 2

½ medium cauliflower, finely chopped
1 leek, finely sliced (optional)
2 tbsp crème fraîche (or 1 tbsp olive oil)

Boil or steam the cauliflower vigorously for 8 minutes, along with the leek, if using. Drain it, and mash it in the same pan with the crème fraîche or olive oil and some salt and freshly ground black pepper.

- **CALORIES** 140
- PROTEIN 5G
- FAT 1G
- FIBRE 4G
- CARBS 4G

White bean or chickpea mash

Serves 2

1 400g tin white beans (e.g. butterbeans, cannelini or chickpeas), rinsed and drained
1 tbsp crème fraîche
2 tbsp olive oil
1 garlic clove, squeezed (optional)
Zest of half a lemon
Salt and pepper to taste

Simmer the beans or chickpeas in 1-2 tbsp water for about 10 minutes to soften them. Add the crème fraîche, olive oil, garlic and lemon zest to the pan and cook the mixture on a medium heat for a few more minutes, then mash it well and season to taste.

- **CALORIES** 290
- PROTEIN 11G
- FAT 17G
- FIBRE 8G
- CARBS 24G

Swede or celeriac mash

Serves 2

½ medium celeriac, peeled and chopped
1 leek, finely sliced (optional)
2 tbsp crème fraîche

Boil the veg vigorously for 10 minutes. Drain it, and mash it in the same pan with the crème fraîche and salt and freshly ground black pepper.

- **CALORIES** 110
- PROTEIN 2G
- FAT 10G
- FIBRE 4G
- CARBS 3G

Green lentils

You can use lentils from a tin for convenience, but cooked from scratch they tend to have better texture and flavour.

Serves 2

1 tbsp olive oil
½ small onion, diced
80g dried green lentils
1 garlic clove, diced (optional)
½ tbsp balsamic vinegar (optional)
200-300ml chicken or vegetable stock

Gently fry the onion for a few minutes in the olive oil, then add the lentils and the garlic, if using, and simmer for 2 more minutes, stirring frequently. Add the balsamic vinegar and the stock (to cover the lentils by about 1½ cm) and simmer for 15 minutes with the lid on. Add a dash of extra water if they are getting dry. Turn the heat off and leave them to steam for a further 10 minutes with the lid on. (Or, if there is still plenty of fluid, continue to simmer gently with the lid off for 5 minutes or so until it has reduced.)

- **CALORIES** 170
- PROTEIN 10G
- FAT 6G
- FIBRE 4G
- CARBS 21G

Cauliflower rice
(see page 98)

Courgetti
(See guilt-free spaghetti, page 107)

Quinoa
(see page 99)

Resistant brown rice
(see page 98)

Konjac noodles

Konjac noodles are made from yam and contain remarkably few calories. There are lots of varieties available on the internet or in large supermarkets (though they are more expensive than usual noodles). They come ready-cooked in a packet and are best rinsed before use. They have a slightly rubbery texture but no particular flavour of their own so they work best when mixed with strong flavours such as in stir-fries, oriental salads or soups.

Cabbage 'noodles'

This can be used as a base for a stir-fry instead of noodles or rice or with a pasta sauce.

Serves 2

½ small cabbage, halved lengthwise, tough core removed and leaves very finely sliced
Dash of olive oil

Steam, boil or microwave the cabbage, so that it is tender but still slightly crunchy. Toss it in the oil and season it with freshly ground black pepper.

- **CALORIES** 70
- PROTEIN 3G
- FAT 4G
- FIBRE 5G
- CARBS 8G

Tips for when you are eating out

- Dump the burger bun, even if it involves scraping the relish back onto the burger.
- Ask to swap the chips for another portion of veg.
- If you have a salad, ask for the dressing on the side so you can choose how much you add. Many restaurant-made dressings are overly sweet.
- Choose the starter and main course and skip the pudding. If you can't resist, ask for extra spoons so you can share with someone else. You get to enjoy the taste, but don't have too much.
- If you have wine, ask the waiter not to top up your glass until it's empty. Alternate sips with water. Ideally avoid alcohol altogether while you're on the diet as this gives your liver a better chance of helping to reduce blood sugars.
- Avoid ordering battered or deep-fried food. Have extra vegetables and greens instead.

What to drink

If you have grown used to squash or cordials, or any other kind of sweetened drink, it can be hard at first to make the switch to water, but I can assure you that your taste buds will adjust and you will soon find sugary drinks far too sweet. You can liven up a jug of water by adding fresh mint leaves, some pieces of cucumber, even a sprig of rosemary. Fizzy water is fine, too – people often find it good to sip when they are hungry.

Herbal and flavoured teas are an excellent way to keep your fluid levels topped up on 800-calorie fast days and can give you a comforting feeling of fullness. (Some people even drink hot water on its own.) You can make extra herbal tea and store it in the fridge to drink cold later.

Remember, too, that milk is back on the agenda. We encourage you to choose semi-skimmed or full-fat milk as it contains more protein and healthy fat-soluble vitamins. Recent studies suggest that people who consume dairy products may have a reduced risk of developing diabetes and even gaining weight. However, remember that milk does contain a fair number of calories.

The Blood Sugar Diet way of life

For those of you who have lost weight and got your blood sugars where you want them to be – congratulations. Hurrah! That is a fantastic achievement and it will have changed your future in a very positive way.

However, take care not to slip back into your old way of eating. To keep the weight off, we recommend that you follow the principles of the low-carbohydrate, Mediterranean-style way of eating outlined in this book for good. You may not need to count the calories so strictly but will still need to monitor portion sizes and avoid snacking.

In our experience, most people find this approach very manageable. We often hear the phrase, 'This is the first diet that I find I can stick to...' And that is the secret of long-term success.

8-Week Meal Planner

Week 1

	Breakfast	Lunch	Dinner	
Mon	Perfect scrambled eggs 210	Smoked fish pate with cucumber 270	Thai red curry with cauliflower rice 300	780
Tue	Yoghurt, nuts and berries 200	Tuna wrap 140	Pork in mustard sauce 290 with broccoli, garlic and anchovy 90	720
Wed	Roasted tomatoes 30 and a boiled egg 80	Halloumi kebabs 430	Michael's fish cakes 130 with mixed leaf salad and parmesan 120	790
Thur	Green eggs and ham 260	Hummus with veg sticks 210	Baked fish with chorizo 270 with Mediterranean veg 130	870
Fri	Yoghurt, nuts and berries 200	Tuna and butterbean salad 410	Bolognese 170 and courgetti 40	820
Sat	Avocado with roasted tomatoes 300	Tzatziki with 2 seeded thin crackers 200	Bulgar wheat risotto 330	830
Sun	Apple and cinnamon porridge 260	Michael's easy roast chicken 260	Miso soup with leftover chicken 200. Option here to skip the soup and have fruit sponge pudding after the roast 360	720 or 880

Week 2

	Breakfast	Lunch	Dinner	
Mon	Scrambled eggs with mushrooms 230	Speedy spicy beans 250	Salmon with lemon and dill 370 with broccoli and asparagus salad 60	910
Tue	Yoghurt, nuts with berries 200	Feta wrap 370	Courgetti with bacon and beans 270	840
Wed	Kipper and tomatoes 230	Paprika chicken kebabs 190	Cauliflower cheese 450	870
Thur	Yoghurt, nuts and berries 200	Greek salad 190	Turkey burgers 180 with red coleslaw 120	690
Fri	Big mushrooms with feta 130	Vietnamese pho 120	Spicy spinach and lentils 320 with spicy roasted cauliflower 220	790
Sat	Pecan chia porridge with raspberries 230	Rainbow salad 120 or option to skip lunch and have the lychee dessert (100) after the korma	Chicken korma with steamed cauli rice 340	690 or 670
Sun	Full English breakfast 330		Moroccan meatballs 390	720

Week 3

	Breakfast	Lunch	Dinner	
Mon	2 simple egg muffins 260	Red pepper soup 150	Courgetti with pesto, goat's cheese and peas 420	830
Tue	2 hard-boiled eggs 160	Chicory with anchovy mayo 170 and seedy flapjack 80	Beef stir-fry 250 with green beans, soy sauce and sesame 120	780
Wed	Porridge with nut butter 310	Red pepper soup 150	Prawn pea salad 300	760
Thur	Big mushrooms with feta 130	Piri piri chicken stick 360	Gammon steak with red cabbage 420	910
Fri	Yoghurt, nuts and berries 200	Tuna wrap 140	Cajun bean burgers 300 with peas and edamame yoghurt 230	870
Sat	Feta wrap 370		Skinny cottage pie 310	680
Sun	Sardines on avocado mash 370	Speedy spicy beans 250	Piri piri chicken 360 with watercress 10 or option to skip lunch and add roasted peaches 90	980 or 710

Week 4

	Breakfast	Lunch	Dinner	
Mon	Cheese and asparagus omelette 290	Lemon prawn kebabs 360	Cajun bean burgers 300 with rocket 10	960
Tue	Kipper and tomatoes 230	Gazpacho 100	Chillied chicken drumsticks 410	740
Wed	Yoghurt, nuts and berries 200	Lentil and feta salad 190	Chinese meatballs 160 with greens with pak choi and oyster sauce 170	720
Thur	Medium oatmeal porridge 290	Chicory with anchovy mayo 170 and seedy flapjack 80	Beef stir-fry 250	790
Fri	Scrambled eggs with smoked salmon 300	Gazpacho 100	Tuna patties 310 with red coleslaw 120	830
Sat	Chia breakfast bircher 340		Lamb hotpot 380 and seedy flapjack 80	800
Sun	Egg baked in avocado 230		Coq au vin 510 with cauli mash 140	880

Week 5

	Breakfast	Lunch	Dinner	
Mon	Perfect scrambled eggs 210	Ploughmans on a stick 400	Chilli squid 160 with rocket and tomato salad 50	820
Tue	Yoghurt, nuts and berries 200	Tuna wrap 140	Chickpea chilli 270 with dollop of creme fraiche 90	700
Wed	Kipper and tomatoes 230	Chicken lime laksa 330	Courgetti puttanesca 160	720
Thur	Green eggs and ham 260	Greek salad 190	Salmon with ginger 210 with green beans, soy sauce and seasme 120	780
Fri	Yoghurt, nuts and berries 200	Chicken lime laksa 330	Beetroot, fig salad 210	740
Sat	Apple and cinnamon porridge 260	Seedy flapjack 80	Spanish chicken with chorizo 540	880
Sun	Avocado with roasted tomatoes 300	Chicory with anchovy mayo 170 or option to skip lunch and have almond pancakes (170) after goulash	Hungarian goulash 350 with kimchi 80	900 or 900

Week 6

	Breakfast	Lunch	Dinner	
Mon	Scrambled eggs with mushrooms 230	Tomato, ham and lentil soup 440	Seafood courgetti 230	900
Tue	Yoghurt, nuts and berries 200	Chinese tofu kebabs 230	Thai red curry with cauli rice 300	730
Wed	Kipper and tomatoes 230	Celeriac and apple soup 320	Chicken drumsticks with garlic crust 440	990
Thur	Yoghurt, nuts and berries 200	Japanese omelette 270	Pork in mustard sauce 290 with greens 30	790
Fri	Big mushrooms with feta 130	Feta wrap 370	Michael's Thai fish cakes 130 with mixed leaf salad and Parmesan 120	750
Sat	Pecan chia porridge with raspberries 230	Smoked fish pate with cucumber 270	Chicken and mushroom pie 250	750
Sun	Full English breakfast 330	Chickpea flatbread 110	Chilli con carne 260 with celeriac mash 110	810

Week 7

	Breakfast	Lunch	Dinner	
Mon	2 hard-boiled eggs 160	Red pepper soup 150	Spicy spinach and lentils 320 with roasted cauliflower 130	760
Tue	2 simple egg muffins 260	Tzatziki with veg sticks 140	Salmon with lemon and dill 370 with broccoli and asparagus salad 60	830
Wed	Porridge with nut butter 310	Red pepper soup 150	Turkey burger 180 with Mediterranean veg 130	770
Thur	Roasted tomatoes 30 with a boiled egg 80	Feta wrap 370	Chicken biriani 390	870
Fri	Yoghurt, nuts and berries 200	Paprika chicken kebabs 190	Courgetti with goat's cheese, pesto and peas 420	810
Sat	Avocado and feta wrap 370	Tzatziki with veg sticks 140 or option to skip lunch and have the lychee dessert after the lasagne 100	Aubergine lasagne 200	710 or 670
Sun	Sardines on avocado mash 370	Rainbow salad 120	Lamb tagine 420	910

Week 8

	Breakfast	Lunch	Dinner	
Mon	Cheese and asparagus omelette 290	Hummus with veg sticks 210	Cajun bean burgers 300 with mixed leaf salad and Parmesan salad 120	920
Tue	Kipper and tomatoes 230	Vietnamese pho 120	Courgetti with tomato meatballs 390	740
Wed	Yoghurt, nuts and berries 200	Poached eggs with spinach 290	Watercress orange and sardine salad 320	810
Thur	Medium oatmeal porridge 290	Vietnamese pho 120	Indian-spiced prawns 190 with spicy roast cauliflower 220	820
Fri	Scrambled eggs with smoked salmon 300	Tuna and butterbean salad 410	Miso soup 90	800
Sat	Chia breakfast bircher 340		Chinese duck pancakes 340 with greens beans, soy sauce and sesame 120	800
Sun	Egg baked in avocado 230	Garlicky aubergine with veg sticks 90	No pasta lasagne 500	820

Index

5:2 diet 7, 10, 199

alcohol 22, 198
almonds
  almond pancakes with cherries 186
  baked spiced apple with nuts 195
  fruit sponge pudding 193
  Parmesan crisps 76
anchovies
  anchovy mayo 173
  broccoli with garlic and anchovy 168
  chicory with anchovy mayo 114
  puttanesca courgetti 110
  roasted red pepper with anchovies 80
apples
  apple and cinnamon porridge 34
  baked spiced apple with nuts 195
  celeriac and apple soup 62
  crunchy red coleslaw with minute steak 119
  gammon steak with red cabbage 152
  healthy ploughmans 75
  ploughmans on a stick 58
apricots
  lamb tagine 139
  pumpkin pudding with crunchy nut topping 188
  roasted 194
  turkey burgers 85
artichokes
  bulgar wheat risotto with chicken and artichokes 129
  halloumi kebabs 58
asparagus
  beef stir-fry with asparagus and sesame seeds 101
  broccoli and asparagus salad 160
  cheese and asparagus omelette 55
  lemon prawn kebabs 56
aubergines
  roasted garlicky aubergine mash 164
  roasted Mediterranean veg 167
  skinny aubergine 'lasagne' 146
avocados
  and feta bash 31
  guacamole 73
  lentil, carrot and avocado salad 118
  with pre-baked tomatoes 31
  sardines on avocado mash 41
  taco lettuce wraps 48–9

bacon
  bacon and broccoli fry-up 53
  carbonara courgetti 110
  cauliflower cheese 83
  coq au vin 142
  courgetti with bacon and beans 108
  egg muffins 42
  full English breakfast 45
  pancetta, broccoli and tomato gratin 151
beans
  beef stir-fry with asparagus and sesame seeds 101
  Cajun-spiced bean burgers 84
  chicken lime laksa 63
  chickpea chilli 104
  chilli con carne 125
  chocolate kidney bean cake 189
  courgetti with bacon and beans 108
  green beans with soy sauce and sesame seeds 170
  runner beans with halloumi 54
  Spanish chicken with chorizo and beans 141
  speedy spicy beans 54
  spring greens with garlic and cannellini beans 170
  Thai red curry 132
  tuna, artichoke and butterbean salad 51
  white bean mash 196
beansprouts
  cabbage stir-fried Chinese style 169
  Vietnamese pho 65
beef
  chilli con carne 125
  courgetti with tomato meatballs 109
  crunchy red coleslaw with minute steak 119
  easy bolognese 124
  Hungarian goulash 140
  Moroccan meatballs in tomato sauce 135
  no-pasta beef 'lasagne' 125
  skinny cottage pie 144
  stir-fry with asparagus and sesame seeds 101
beetroot
  rainbow salad 162
  roasted beetroot and fig salad 119
  spiced purple veg 160
berries
  almond pancakes with cherries 186
  berry coulis or 'jam' 189
  Greek yoghurt with nuts, seeds and berries 33
  pecan chia porridge with raspberries 36
  seedy flapjacks 76
black pudding, full English breakfast 45
blood sugar, glycaemic index/load (GI/GL) 15
blood sugar diet
  precautions 17
  preparation 18
  principles 8, 9–10, 12, 22–3
blueberries
  rainbow salad 162
  seedy flapjacks 76
bolognese, easy 124
Brazil nuts
  pear and Brazil nut chocolate brownies 191
  savoury butter 75
bread
  chickpea flatbread 183
  flour 180
  reduction 12
  seeded spelt and rye 181
  types 178
  wholegrain soda 180
breakfast
  advanced prep 39
  blood sugar diet 24
  full English 45
broccoli
  and asparagus salad 160
  bacon and broccoli fry-up 53
  with garlic and anchovy 168
  pancetta, broccoli and tomato gratin 151
brownies, pear and Brazil nut 191
bulgar wheat
  basic cooking method 99
  risotto with chicken and artichokes 129
  tabbouleh with pine nuts 159
burgers
  Cajun-spiced bean 84
  turkey 85
buttermilk dressing 176
butternut squash
  chicken lime laksa 63
  lamb tagine 139
  low-carb lamb hotpot 149
  piri piri chicken sticks 60
  roasted red pepper and squash soup 68

cabbage
  chicken and mushroom 'pie' 147
  chickpeas with Indian-spiced stir-fried greens 102
  crunchy red coleslaw 158
  crunchy red coleslaw with minute steak 119
  gammon steak with red cabbage 152
  Japanese omelette 55
  no-pasta beef 'lasagne' 125
  'noodles' 198
  pickled cabbage (kimchi) 161
  prawn and tuna fried rice 111
  spiced purple veg 160
  spring greens with garlic and cannellini beans 170
  stir-fried cabbage with peppered mackerel 104
  stir-fried Chinese style 169
Cajun-spiced bean burgers 84
cake, chocolate kidney bean 189
carbohydrates 12, 15
carbonara courgetti 110
carrots
  coq au vin 142
  crunchy red coleslaw 158
  crunchy red coleslaw with minute steak 119
  easy bolognese 124
  easy roast chicken with garlic and thyme 155
  Hungarian goulash 140
  lentil, carrot and avocado salad 118

low-carb lamb hotpot 149
rainbow salad 162
cauliflower
cauliflower cheese 83
cauliflower rice 98
chicken and mushroom 'pie' 147
chicken korma 131
creamy skinny kedgeree 97
easy roast chicken with garlic and thyme 155
mash 196
prawn and tuna fried rice 111
simple roasted 165
skinny cottage pie 144
spicy roasted 165
celeriac
Cajun-spiced bean burgers 84
celeriac and apple soup 62
creamy fish bake 145
low-carb pizza 136
mash 197
cheese
avocados and feta bash 31
cauliflower cheese 83
cheese and asparagus omelette 55
chicken and mushroom 'pie' 147
courgetti with pesto, goat's cheese and peas 107
egg muffins 42
Greek salad 51
ham and cheese omelette 42
healthy ploughmans 75
lentil and feta salad 50
low-carb pizza 136
mixed leaf salad with rocket and shaved Parmesan 158
mushrooms with feta 30
no-pasta beef 'lasagne' 125
pancetta, broccoli and tomato gratin 151
Parmesan crisps 76
pear, hazelnut and goat's cheese salad 114
ploughmans on a stick 58
quiche in a dish 86
roasted beetroot and fig salad 119
runner beans with halloumi 54
skinny aubergine 'lasagne' 146
skinny cottage pie 144
taco lettuce wrap 49
turkey burgers 85
cherries, almond pancakes with cherries 186
chia seeds
baked spiced apple with nuts 195
berry coulis or 'jam' 189
chia breakfast bircher 38
chia kulfi 184
extra-filling porridge with nut butter 35
low-sugar sweet chilli sauce 175
pecan chia porridge with raspberries 36
thin seeded crackers 75
chicken
biriani with cauli rice 105
bulgar wheat risotto with chicken and artichokes 129
chicken and mushroom 'pie' 147
chicken lime laksa 63
coq au vin 142
drumsticks 2 ways 88
easy roast chicken with garlic and thyme 155
korma 131
lazy chicken and spicy lentils 154
paprika chicken kebab 59
piri piri chicken sticks 60
satay chicken kebabs 61
Spanish chicken with chorizo and beans 141
Thai red curry 132
wrapped in Parma ham 89
chickpea flatbread 183
chickpeas
chickpea chilli 104
hummus 71
with Indian-spiced stir-fried greens 102
mash 196
Moroccan spiced chickpea salad 117
spicy tuna fish patties 90
chicory
with anchovy mayo 114
pear, hazelnut and goat's cheese salad 114
chilli
chilli squid with lentils 93
low-sugar sweet chilli sauce 175
red salsa 176
scrambled eggs 27
chilli con carne 125
Chinese duck with green 'pancakes' 136
Chinese pork meatballs 85
Chinese tofu kebabs 60
chocolate
chocolate kidney bean cake 189
pear and Brazil nut chocolate brownies 191
chorizo
baked fish and chorizo parcels 152
Spanish chicken with chorizo and beans 141
coconut milk, chia breakfast bircher 38
coconut oil 15–16, 35
chocolate kidney bean cake 189
fruit sponge pudding 193
seedy flapjacks 76
coconut yoghurt 33
coleslaw
crunchy red coleslaw 158
with minute steak 119
coq au vin 142
cottage cheese
egg muffins 42
skinny aubergine 'lasagne' 146
smoked mackerel and mushroom frittata 132
courgettes
paprika chicken kebabs 59
roasted Mediterranean veg 167
salmon with lemon and dill nut crust on roasted veg 94
speedy spicy beans 54
courgetti
with bacon and beans 108
carbonara 110
with pesto, goat's cheese and peas 107
puttanesca 110
with seafood 108
with tomato meatballs 109
crackers, thin seeded 75
cucumber
Chinese duck with green 'pancakes' 136
gazpacho 68
Greek salad 51
Moroccan spiced chickpea salad 117
raitha 72
smoked fish paté 73
tabbouleh with pine nuts 159
tzatziki 72
curry
chicken biriani with cauli rice 105
chicken korma 131
chicken lime laksa 63
Indian spiced prawns 91
Thai red curry 132

dairy alternatives 33
dairy products 13, 33, 199 *see also* yoghurt
dates
baked spiced apple with nuts 195
chocolate kidney bean cake 189
fruit sponge pudding 193
orange and pistachio cupcakes 185
pear and Brazil nut chocolate brownies 191
roasted peaches 194
seedy flapjacks 76
diabetes 7, 17
dips
guacamole 73
hummus 71
raitha 72
smoked fish paté 73
tzatziki 72
doctor's support 17
dressings
buttermilk dressing 176
French vinaigrette 173
garlic and lemon yoghurt dressing 175
mayo 4 ways 172–3
restaurant tips 198
yoghurt and mustard dressing 175
drinks 22, 199
duck, Chinese duck with green 'pancakes' 136

eggs
baked in avocado 43
boiled 39
carbonara courgetti 110
creamy skinny kedgeree 97
egg muffins 42
full English breakfast 45
mushroom omelette 28
poached with spinach and pine nuts 29
quiche in a dish 86
scrambled with variations 27
simple omelette 28

smoked mackerel and mushroom frittata 132

fast days 7, 22–3, 199
fat, visceral 7, 16
fats, dietary 9, 13, 15–16
fennel
crunchy red coleslaw 158
piri piri chicken 141
roasted Mediterranean veg 167
feta
avocados and feta bash 31
Greek salad 51
lentil and feta salad 50
mushrooms with feta 30
roasted beetroot and fig salad 119
taco lettuce wrap with avocado 49
figs
chia breakfast bircher 38
roasted beetroot and fig salad 119
fish
baked fish and chorizo parcels 152
broccoli with garlic and anchovy 168
chicory with anchovy mayo 114
creamy fish bake 145
creamy skinny kedgeree 97
eggs baked in avocado 43
kipper and tomatoes 29
prawn and tuna fried rice 111
puttanesca courgetti 110
roasted red pepper with anchovies 80
salmon with coconut and chilli 96
salmon with ginger 96
salmon with lemon and dill nut crust on roasted veg 94
sardines on avocado mash 41
smoked fish paté 73
smoked mackerel and mushroom frittata 132
smoked salmon scrambled eggs 27
spicy tuna fish patties 90
stir-fried cabbage with peppered mackerel 104
taco lettuce wraps 48–9
Thai fish cakes 126
tuna, artichoke and butterbean salad 51
watercress, orange and sardine salad 112
flapjacks, seedy flapjacks 76
flavour boosts 23
flour 180
French vinaigrette 173
frittata, smoked mackerel and mushroom 132
fruit *see also* specific fruit
fruit sponge pudding 193
spicy fruit porridge 36
sugar levels 13, 192

gammon steak with red cabbage 152
gazpacho 68
glycaemic index/load (GI/GL) 15
goals 16
grapefruit, lychee and pink grapefruit salad 193
Greek salad 51
Greek yoghurt with nuts, seeds and berries 33
guacamole 73
gut bacteria 33, 101, 114

halloumi
kebabs 58
runner beans with halloumi 54
turkey burgers 85
ham
chicken wrapped in Parma ham 89
gammon steak with red cabbage 152
green eggs and ham 27
ham and cheese omelette 42
ploughmans on a stick 58
tomato, ham and lentil soup 66
hummus 71
taco lettuce wrap with roast peppers and nuts 49
Hungarian goulash 140
hunger signals 9, 15, 22

Indian spiced prawns 91
insulin 17
inulin 101, 114

Japanese omelette 55

kebabs
Chinese tofu 60
halloumi 58
lemon prawn 56
paprika chicken 59
piri piri chicken sticks 60
ploughmans on a stick 58
satay chicken 61
spiced lamb 59
kedgeree, creamy skinny 97
kimchi 161
kipper and tomatoes 29
konjac noodles 198
konjac rice 99
kulfi, quick chia 184

lamb
garlic and rosemary fried lamb 130
low-carb lamb hotpot 149
Moroccan meatballs in tomato sauce 135
spiced lamb kebabs 59
tagine 139
'lasagne,' skinny aubergine 146
leeks, chicken and mushroom 'pie' 147
lemon prawn kebabs 56
lentils
chickpeas with Indian-spiced stir-fried greens 102
chilli squid with lentils 93
green lentils 197
lazy chicken and spicy lentils 154
lentil and feta salad 50
lentil, carrot and avocado salad 118
spicy spinach and lentils 81
spicy stuffed red pepper 123
tomato, ham and lentil soup 66
lettuce *see also* salads
Chinese duck with green 'pancakes' 136
taco lettuce wrap 4 ways 48–9
low-fat foods 22, 33
lunch 46
lychee and pink grapefruit salad 193

mackerel
smoked fish paté 73
smoked mackerel and mushroom frittata 132
stir-fried cabbage with peppered mackerel 104
margaric acid 13
mayo 4 ways 172–3
meatballs
Chinese pork meatballs 85
courgetti with tomato meatballs 109
Moroccan meatballs in tomato sauce 135
medications 17
Mediterranean diet 8, 10, 12–13
milk 199
miso soup 67
Moroccan meatballs in tomato sauce 135
Moroccan spiced chickpea salad 117
motivation 16
mushrooms
bacon and broccoli fry-up 53
chicken and mushroom 'pie' 147
chickpea chilli 104
chilli con carne 125
coq au vin 142
egg muffins 42
with feta 30
full English breakfast 45
lazy chicken and spicy lentils 154
omelette 28
roasted red pepper with anchovies 80
scrambled eggs 27
skinny aubergine 'lasagne' 146
smoked mackerel and mushroom frittata 132
spiced lamb kebabs 59

noodles
konjac 198
Vietnamese pho 65
nutrition 23
nuts
avocados and feta bash 31
baked spiced apple with nuts 195
chia breakfast bircher 38
chia kulfi 184
crunchy red coleslaw 158
extra-filling porridge with nut butter 35
fruit sponge pudding 193
Greek yoghurt with nuts, seeds and berries 33
home-made pesto 177
orange and pistachio cupcakes 185
Parmesan crisps 76
pear and Brazil nut chocolate brownies 191
pear, hazelnut and goat's cheese salad 114
pecan chia porridge with raspberries 36
poached eggs with spinach and pine nuts 29

pumpkin pudding with crunchy nut topping 188
roasted peaches 194
roasted red pepper with anchovies 80
salmon with lemon and dill nut crust on roasted veg 94
savoury Brazil nut butter 75
snacking 74
tabbouleh with pine nuts 159
taco lettuce wrap with roast peppers and hummus 49
toasting 39

oats 34 *see also* porridge
chia breakfast bircher 38
seedy flapjacks 76
wholegrain soda bread 180
olive oil 15, 51
olives
Greek salad 51
low-carb pizza 136
puttanesca courgetti 110
Spanish chicken with chorizo and beans 141
omelettes
cheese and asparagus 55
Japanese 55
mushroom 28
simple 28
onions
chicken biriani with cauli rice 105
creamy skinny kedgeree 97
easy roast chicken with garlic and thyme 155
Greek salad 51
lamb tagine 139
paprika chicken kebabs 59
ploughmans on a stick 58
roasted Mediterranean veg 167
salmon with lemon and dill nut crust on roasted veg 94
speedy spicy beans 54
spiced purple veg 160
spicy stuffed red pepper 123
oranges
orange and pistachio cupcakes 185
watercress, orange and sardine salad 112

pak choi with oyster sauce 169
pancakes, almond pancakes with cherries 186
pancetta, broccoli and tomato gratin 151
paprika chicken kebab 59
Parmesan crisps 76
passion fruit
chia breakfast bircher 38
instant creamy passion fruit pudding 184
pasta substitutes 12, 107
paté, smoked fish 73
peaches, roasted 194
pears
pear and Brazil nut chocolate brownies 191
pear, hazelnut and goat's cheese salad 114
peas
courgetti with pesto, goat's cheese and peas 107
peas and edamame with yoghurt and lime dressing 167
prawn, pea and spring onion salad 118
pecan chia porridge with raspberries 36
peppers
bulgar wheat risotto with chicken and artichokes 129
cauliflower cheese 83
chicken lime laksa 63
chickpea chilli 104
chilli con carne 125
Chinese tofu kebabs 60
gazpacho 68
halloumi kebabs 58
Hungarian goulash 140
lamb tagine 139
low-sugar sweet chilli sauce 175
piri piri chicken 141
prawn and tuna fried rice 111
rainbow salad 162
red salsa 176
roasted Mediterranean veg 167
roasted red pepper and squash soup 68
roasted red pepper with anchovies 80
salmon with ginger 96
salmon with lemon and dill nut crust on roasted veg 94
skinny aubergine 'lasagne' 146
speedy spicy beans 54
spiced lamb kebabs 59
spicy stuffed red pepper 123
spicy tuna fish patties 90
taco lettuce wrap with hummus and nuts 49
Thai red curry 132
tomato, ham and lentil soup 66
pesto, home-made 177
pine nuts see nuts
piri piri chicken 141
piri piri chicken sticks 60
pizza, low-carb 136
ploughmans, healthy 75
ploughmans on a stick 58
pork
Chinese pork meatballs 85
pork steaks in mustard sauce 128
porridge
advanced prep 39
apple and cinnamon porridge 34
extra-filling with nut butter 35
medium oatmeal 35
pecan chia porridge with raspberries 36
spicy fruit 36
prawns
Indian spiced prawns 91
prawn and tuna fried rice 111
prawn, pea and spring onion salad 118
Vietnamese pho 65
protein 13
pumpkin pudding with crunchy nut topping 188
puttanesca courgetti 110

quiche in a dish 86
quinoa
basic cooking method 99
garlic and rosemary fried lamb 130
Moroccan spiced chickpea salad 117

radishes, rainbow salad 162
rainbow salad 162
raitha 72
raspberries, pecan chia porridge with raspberries 36
red salsa 176
restaurant tips 198
rhubarb, roasted with ginger 194
rice substitutes 12, 98–9
risotto, bulgar wheat with chicken and artichokes 129
runner beans with halloumi 54

salads
Greek 51
lentil and feta 50
lentil, carrot and avocado 118
lychee and pink grapefruit 193
mixed leaf salad with rocket and shaved Parmesan 158
Moroccan spiced chickpea 117
prawn, pea and spring onion 118
rainbow 162
roasted beetroot and fig 119
tuna, artichoke and butterbean 51
watercress, orange and sardine 112
salmon
with coconut and chilli 96
with ginger 96
with lemon and dill nut crust on roasted veg 94
smoked salmon scrambled eggs 27
taco lettuce wrap with avocado 48
salt 22
sardines
sardines on avocado mash 41
watercress, orange and sardine salad 112
satay chicken kebabs 61
satiety 9, 13
sauces
home-made pesto 177
low-sugar sweet chilli sauce 175
red salsa 176
sausages, full English breakfast 45
seafood *see also* fish; prawns
chilli squid with lentils 93
courgetti with seafood 108
seeds *see also* chia seeds
beef stir-fry with asparagus and sesame seeds 101
Greek yoghurt with nuts, seeds and berries 33
green beans with soy sauce and sesame seeds 170
seeded spelt and rye bread 181
seedy flapjacks 76
thin seeded crackers 75
toasting 39
wholegrain soda bread 180
skinny cottage pie 144

smoked mackerel
  smoked fish paté 73
  smoked mackerel and mushroom frittata 132
smoked salmon
  eggs baked in avocado 43
  scrambled eggs 27
  taco lettuce wrap with avocado 48
snacks 16, 46
soups 22
  celeriac and apple 62
  chicken lime laksa 63
  gazpacho 68
  miso 67
  roasted red pepper and squash 68
  tomato, ham and lentil 66
  Vietnamese pho 65
Spanish chicken with chorizo and beans 141
spinach
  chicken lime laksa 63
  creamed spinach 167
  egg muffins 42
  full English breakfast 45
  green eggs and ham 27
  Indian spiced prawns 91
  mushrooms with feta 30
  no-pasta beef 'lasagne' 125
  poached eggs with spinach and pine nuts 29
  quiche in a dish 86
  skinny aubergine 'lasagne' 146
  smoked mackerel and mushroom frittata 132
  spicy spinach and lentils 81
spring greens with garlic and cannellini beans 170
squid, chilli squid with lentils 93
store cupboard 18–20
sugar 12, 192
swede mash 197
sweeteners, artificial 15, 192
Swiss chard stir-fried with garlic 168

tabbouleh with pine nuts 159
taco lettuce wrap 4 ways 48–9
teas 199
Thai fish cakes 126
Thai red curry 132
tofu, Chinese tofu kebabs 60
tomatoes
  advanced prep 39
  avocados with pre-baked tomatoes 31
  baked fish and chorizo parcels 152
  chickpea chilli 104
  courgetti with tomato meatballs 109
  easy bolognese 124
  full English breakfast 45
  gazpacho 68
  Greek salad 51
  Hungarian goulash 140
  Indian spiced prawns 91
  kipper and tomatoes 29
  lemon prawn kebabs 56
  Moroccan meatballs in tomato sauce 135
  Moroccan spiced chickpea salad 117
  pancetta, broccoli and tomato gratin 151
  piri piri chicken 141
  piri piri chicken sticks 60
  puttanesca courgetti 110
  rainbow salad 162
  roasted Mediterranean veg 167
  roasted red pepper with anchovies 80
  skinny aubergine 'lasagne' 146
  skinny cottage pie 144
  Spanish chicken with chorizo and beans 141
  spring greens with garlic and cannellini beans 170
  tabbouleh with pine nuts 159
  taco lettuce wrap with tuna 49
  tomato, ham and lentil soup 66
  tuna, artichoke and butterbean salad 51
topping suggestions 177
treats 178
tuna
prawn and tuna fried rice 111
spicy tuna fish patties 90
taco lettuce wrap with tomato salsa 49
tuna, artichoke and butterbean salad 51
turkey burgers 85
tzatziki 72

vegetables *see also* specific vegetables
  Mediterranean diet 12–13
  roasted Mediterranean veg 167
  salmon with lemon and dill nut crust on roasted veg 94
  spiced purple veg 160
Vietnamese pho 65
vinegar 13
visceral fat 7
vitamins 23

water 22, 199
watercress
  rainbow salad 162
  watercress, orange and sardine salad 112
weight loss, diabetes prevention 7–8
white bean mash 196
wine, restaurant tips 198

yoghurt
  garlic and lemon yoghurt dressing 175
  Greek yoghurt with nuts, seeds and berries 33
  peas and edamame with yoghurt and lime dressing 167
  raitha 72
  tzatziki 72
  yoghurt and mustard dressing 175

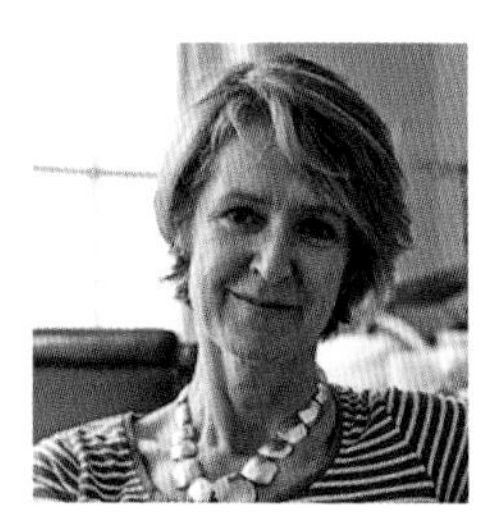

Dr Clare Bailey, wife of Michael Mosley, is a GP who has pioneered the Blood Sugar Diet approach at her surgery in Buckinghamshire. She has four children.

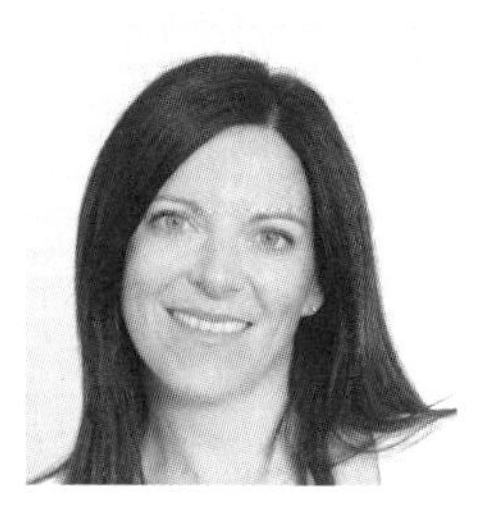

Dr Sarah Schenker is a registered dietitian and nutritionist. She is the nutritional adviser for the bestselling *The Fast Diet Recipe Book* (Short Books, 2013) and regularly contributes to newspapers and magazines including the *Daily Mail*, *Top Sante* and *Glamour* as well as shows including This Morning, Watchdog and on BBC Radio.